Computed tomography
of the human body

AN ATLAS OF NORMAL ANATOMY

Computed tomography of the human body

AN ATLAS OF NORMAL ANATOMY

RALPH J. ALFIDI, M.D.

Head, Department of Hospital Radiology,
Cleveland Clinic, Cleveland, Ohio

JOHN HAAGA, M.D.

Radiologist, Department of Radiology,
Cleveland Clinic, Cleveland, Ohio

MEREDITH WEINSTEIN, M.D.

Head, Division of Cranial CT Scanning,
Cleveland Clinic, Cleveland, Ohio

JACK DeGROOT, M.D., Ph.D.

Professor of Anatomy,
University of California at San Francisco,
San Francisco, California

with 220 illustrations

The C. V. Mosby Company

Saint Louis   1977

Printed in the United States of America

Distributed in Great Britain by Henry Kimpton, London

The C. V. Mosby Company
11830 Westline Industrial Drive, St. Louis, Missouri 63141

Library of Congress Cataloging in Publication Data

Main entry under title:

Computed tomography of the human body.

   Includes index.
   1. Tomography—Atlases. 2. Anatomy, Human—
Atlases. I. Alfidi, Ralph J. [DNLM: 1. Anatomy,
regional atlases. 2. Tomography, computerized axial—
Atlases. QS17 C738]
RC78.7.T6C65   616.07'572   77-7095
ISBN 0-8016-0116-9

TS/U/B 9 8 7 6 5 4 3 2 1

To
our wives, friends, and colleagues,
who made valuable suggestions and urged us on
to the completion of this book

PREFACE

Revolutionary advances in computed tomography (CT) have occurred in a short time. In 1917 Radon, an Austrian mathematician, proved that a three-dimensional object could be reconstructed mathematically from an infinite set of projections. In 1961, using a gamma ray source and a collimated scintillation counter, Olendorf passed a photon beam through an object to measure the attenuation coefficient at the center of rotation. Other investigators who worked in areas closely related to computed tomography as we know it today were Cormack in 1963, Kuhl and Edwards in 1968, and Gordon, Bender, and Herman in 1970.

Godfrey N. Hounsfield, an electronic research engineer at Electrical and Musical Industries in England, developed the first clinically useful CT scanner of the brain. He collaborated with Dr. James Ambrose, a radiologist at Atkinson-Morely Hospital, to make CT scanning of the human brain a reality. Dr. Hounsfield's work began in 1967; on October 1, 1971, the first working CT scanner was installed at Atkinson-Morely Hospital. On April 19, 1972, Dr. Ambrose was able to report clinical results of CT scanning to the Annual Congress of the British Institute of Radiology.

This revolutionary work was followed rapidly by development of the first whole-body scanner by R. S. Ledley in 1974. In 1975, the Ohio Nuclear Corporation developed and introduced the second whole-body scanner. Since that time, some thirty manufacturers have announced that they are in various phases of development of brain and body CT scanners. This extremely rapid development of computed tomography has resulted in a new horizon of imaging techniques that has significantly changed the present and future of both diagnosis and treatment.

This atlas will hopefully provide imaging specialists with the basic groundwork for the study of CT images. The anatomical specimens and corresponding CT images represent state of the art imaging to make the identification of pathological conditions a less cumbersome task than we initially experienced in viewing and learning CT anatomy.

Ralph J. Alfidi, John Haaga, Meredith Weinstein, and Jack DeGroot

ACKNOWLEDGMENTS

The photographic specimens shown in this text were produced through the efforts of Mr. Steven Robinson and Mr. Robert Maynard. Considerable experimentation with CT photography was required before the excellent plates shown became possible. We also wish to express our thanks to Dr. Martha Sucheson for some of the early images that were made. Our special thanks to Dr. Antonio Rodriquez-Antunez for providing funds from his special grant that made it possible to purchase a device which would permit the freezing of entire cadavers. We also wish to express our thanks to the members of the Cleveland Clinic Department of Pathology, Drs. William Hawk and Howard Levin, not only for their cooperation in the use of equipment but for their suggestions as well. We are grateful to Steve Gianelos, Jim Boles, Ellen Dietrick, and Susan Edelman for giving radiologic and technical assistance during the examination preparation of the cadaver specimens. Last, we would be remiss if we did not express thanks to our publisher and to the many radiologists who urged us on in the production of this text.

CONTENTS

Chapter 1

INTRODUCTION

Cross-sectional anatomy of the body, until recently, has been only of peripheral interest to the practicing physician. With the advent of computed tomography (CT), detailed and accurate cross-sectional anatomy has become a necessity. Early in our experience with computed tomography, it became obvious that the cross-sectional anatomy portrayed in anatomical texts did not match the images obtained with CT. Our "conceptualized" localization of the gallbladder, common bile duct, pancreas, third and fourth ventricles, adrenal glands, and the second portion of the duodenum obviously required readjustment.

Countless hours were spent in identifying and reorienting our two-dimensional knowledge of the three-dimensional structure of the body that CT requires. It also is most useful to think of multiple reconstructions in a three-dimensional mental sense. Since we are not yet able to produce three-dimensional images with computed tomography, the most versatile of computers, the brain, must be employed to store and mentally reconstruct this imagery. If we incorrectly reconstruct in our minds the relationship of the kidney to the adrenal, then small adrenal tumors may be missed. We now know that one should attempt to identify the superior mesenteric artery and the crura of the diaphragm in order to differentiate the pancreas from the duodenum. Dilute oral contrast material may be used to help in differentiating the bowel from the pancreas.

VIEWING OF ANATOMICAL SPECIMENS

Originally, CT sections of the brain were viewed as if one were looking from above, with the left side on the viewer's left. This is the conventional manner in which radiographs are viewed. Initial articles on computed tomography of the body showed it viewed in the same fashion, that is, from above. Because of the convention of viewing ultrasound images from below, which was established only a short time ago, it was decided at the Second International Symposium of Computed Tomography to view body sections in the same manner. Either convention has merit. At the present time most cerebral examinations are viewed and photographed from above and most examinations of the body are viewed and photographed from below. This book presents the entire body as viewed from below. It is hoped that in the near future the entire corpus will be viewed in the same fashion and published similarly.

MATERIALS, METHODS, AND TECHNIQUES
Cadavers

Four cadavers (two male, two female) were scanned within 72 hours after death. Contiguous sections of the cadavers were made at 13 mm intervals from the top of the head to the floor of the pelvis. The cadavers were then placed in a freezer maintained at $-25°$ F. After 3 to 4 days the cadavers were completely frozen.

The anatomical sections were made by sectioning the cadavers with a large band saw. The blade of the saw was positioned to match the center of each CT section. The band saw was 2 mm thick. Both the superior and inferior aspects of each of the specimens were photographed. An embalmed cadaver was used to make the anatomical sections of the head at 25 degrees to the orbitomeatal line. The CT sections of the head and neck were selected from patient scans to match the anatomical specimens. Virtually all these patients had 100 ml of iothalamate sodium (CONRAY-400) administered intravenously immediately prior to obtaining the scans. After the administration of contrast material, the white and gray matter of the brain and the major intracerebral vessels could be well defined by CT. These structures could not be well defined on CT scans performed on the cadavers.

The CT sections of the thorax, abdomen, and pelvis were obtained from the matching anatomical section. The CT sections of the thorax, abdomen, and pelvis are a composite of the four cadavers scanned. Most of the sections of the head and body were obtained at 13 mm intervals. Additional sections were inserted in these regions for teaching and illustrative points. It was not always possible to find clinical material exactly in the same plane as the anatomical sections of the head and neck. The CT sections were selected so as to best illustrate the major anatomical structures. Sections were omitted in the superior aspect of the head and in the thorax and lower abdomen where the anatomy did not significantly change from section to section.

Artifacts

Two embalmed cadavers were scanned. Both of these cadavers had gas within the biliary tree and blood vessels of the body. The gas caused objectionable CT artifacts. The attenuation coefficients of the tissues were altered by the embalming fluid. On the CT scans of the embalmed cadavers, the fat planes between the muscles were partially obliterated. The embalmed sections were not used for the body portion of this atlas.

All the cadavers had large pleural effusions present within the chest. There was retraction of pulmonary tissues anteriorly. Fortunately, the relationships of the vascular structures remain ordered, so that this retraction does not interfere with orientation. Artifacts caused by ice crystals are present on many of the anatomical slices. The artifacts caused by these crystals can be seen when a high-resolution black and white film is used. Defrosting the surface of the anatomical specimen does not entirely remove these artifacts.

The artifact visualized in the midoccipital region of the embalmed skull (pp. 5 to 12) was caused by a tube used for embalming.

Photography

The specimens were photographed using a Polaroid MP3 Industrial camera with 135 mm lens. We used Ilford black and white FB-4 film and a D 76 developer. This film was selected after trying several films of different speed resolution and contrast. Black and white film was used to limit the cost of this atlas and because this film could be varied to enhance resolution or contrast. The CT images were photographed directly from the cathode ray tube. A Hasselblad 70 mm camera was used with FB-4 film.

When the CT images were enlarged to a size greater than the 5-inch by 7-inch photograph, undesirable raster lines were produced. Anatomical detail was also lost by this enlargement. Therefore the CT images of the head in Chapter 2 are printed in both large and small format.

Labeling

All structures have been labeled using the commonly accepted medical terminology rather than the somewhat archaic terminology found in earlier classic anatomy texts. The labeling of the anatomical specimens was dictated by their visibility in the CT image. Where structures in the CT image were impossible to define against the background, it was considered useless to attempt to portray anatomical structures that were either too small to visualize or of insufficient difference in attenuation coefficient to be shown.

CT apparatus

The clinical material used for the CT scans of the head and base of the skull was obtained on a prototype model of the Ohio Nuclear Delta 25 Scanner. The matrix is 256 by 256. To decrease the amount of overlapping white and gray matter within each section, 8 mm thick sections were used to examine the brain. Five mm thick sections were used in the orbit to maximize spatial resolution.

The neck and body CT sections were performed on a prototype model of the Ohio Nuclear Delta 50 Scanner. CT sections of the body were obtained using a 13 mm thickness.

Chapter 2

HEAD AND NECK

MEREDITH WEINSTEIN
JACK DeGROOT

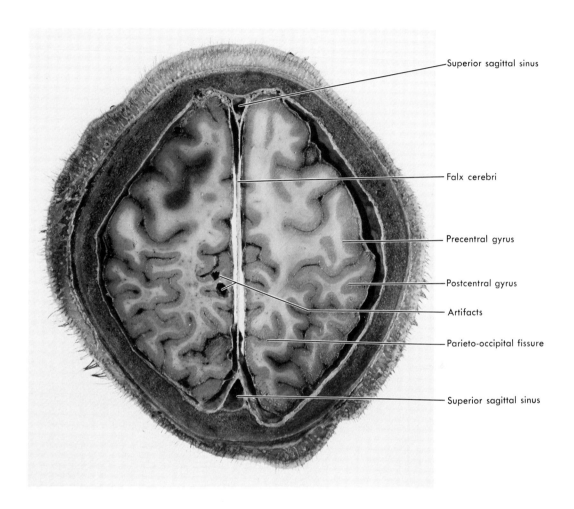

Superior sagittal sinus

Falx cerebri

Precentral gyrus

Postcentral gyrus

Artifacts

Parieto-occipital fissure

Superior sagittal sinus

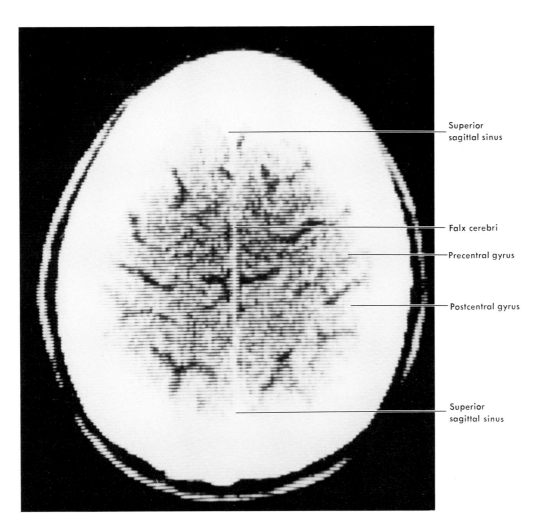

Superior sagittal sinus

Falx cerebri

Precentral gyrus

Postcentral gyrus

Superior sagittal sinus

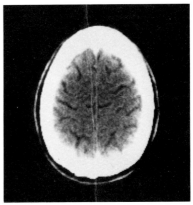

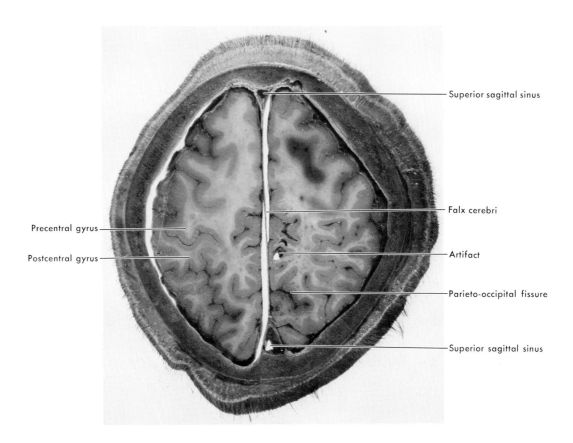

Precentral gyrus

Postcentral gyrus

Superior sagittal sinus

Falx cerebri

Artifact

Parieto-occipital fissure

Superior sagittal sinus

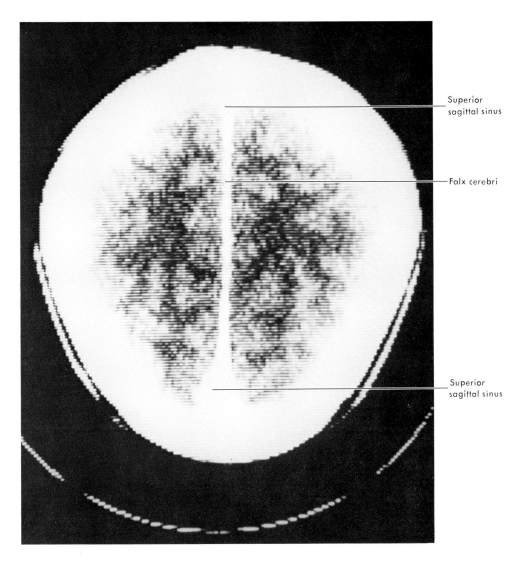

Superior
sagittal sinus

Falx cerebri

Superior
sagittal sinus

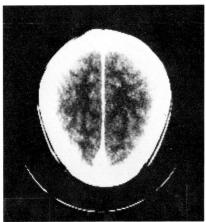

Computed tomography of the human body

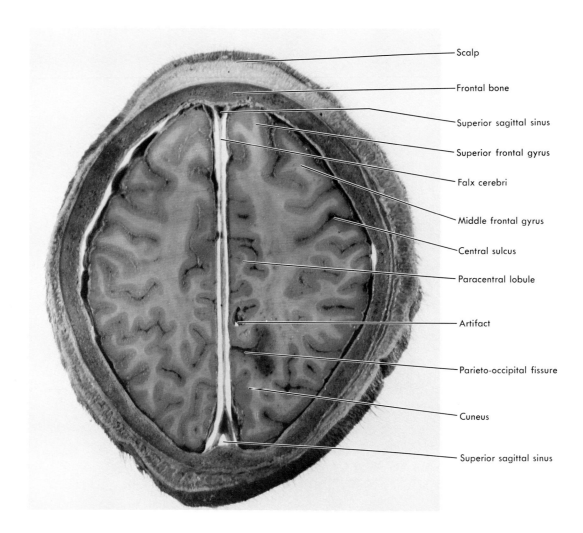

Scalp

Frontal bone

Superior sagittal sinus

Superior frontal gyrus

Falx cerebri

Middle frontal gyrus

Central sulcus

Paracentral lobule

Artifact

Parieto-occipital fissure

Cuneus

Superior sagittal sinus

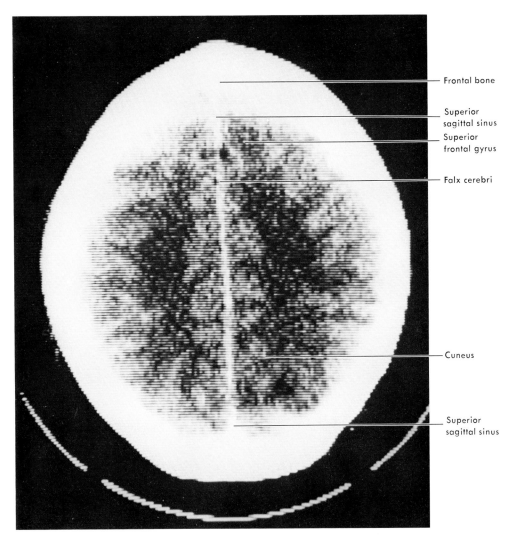

Frontal bone

Superior
sagittal sinus

Superior
frontal gyrus

Falx cerebri

Cuneus

Superior
sagittal sinus

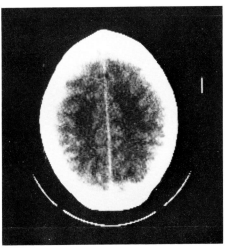

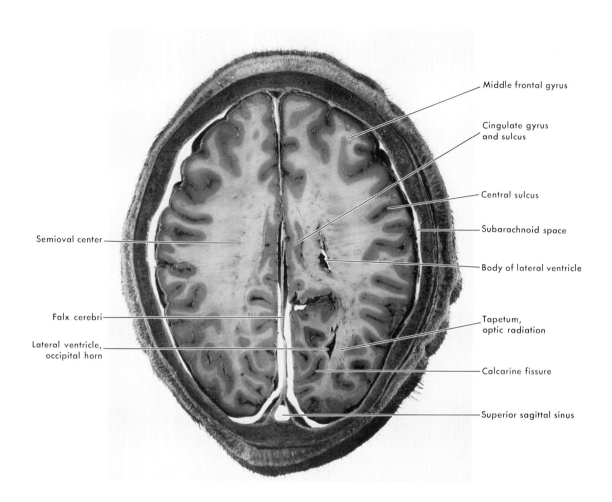

Middle frontal gyrus

Cingulate gyrus
and sulcus

Central sulcus

Subarachnoid space

Semioval center

Body of lateral ventricle

Falx cerebri

Tapetum,
optic radiation

Lateral ventricle,
occipital horn

Calcarine fissure

Superior sagittal sinus

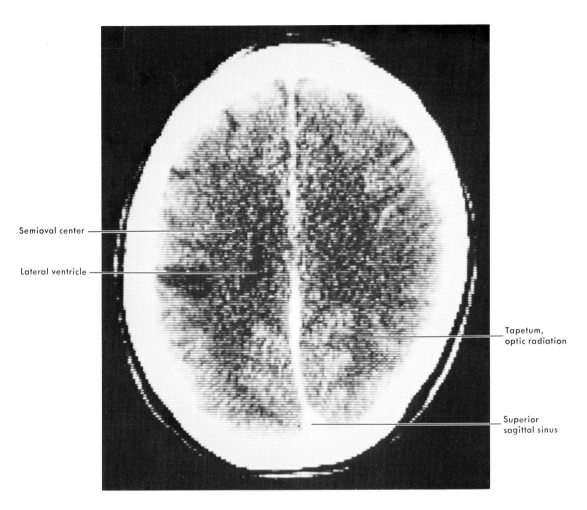

Semioval center

Lateral ventricle

Tapetum,
optic radiation

Superior
sagittal sinus

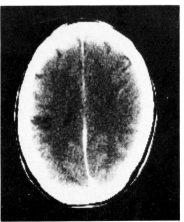

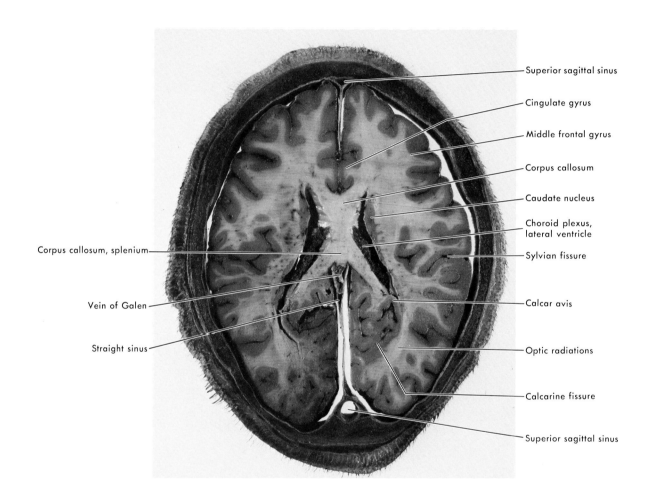

Superior sagittal sinus

Cingulate gyrus

Middle frontal gyrus

Corpus callosum

Caudate nucleus

Choroid plexus, lateral ventricle

Sylvian fissure

Calcar avis

Optic radiations

Calcarine fissure

Superior sagittal sinus

Corpus callosum, splenium

Vein of Galen

Straight sinus

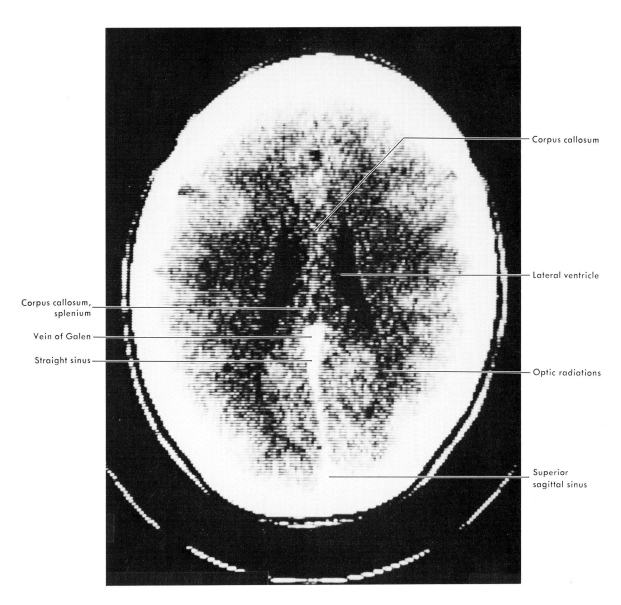

Corpus callosum

Lateral ventricle

Corpus callosum,
splenium

Vein of Galen

Straight sinus

Optic radiations

Superior
sagittal sinus

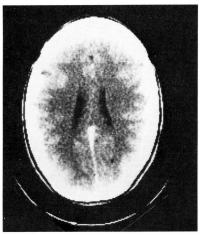

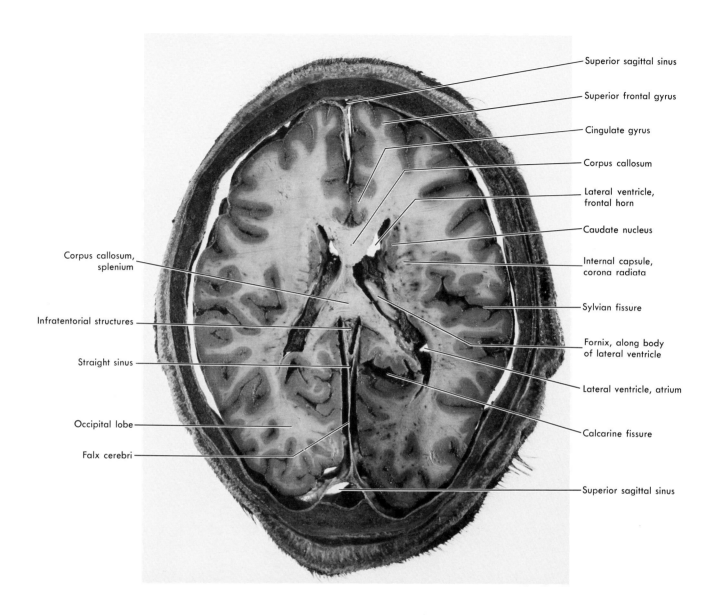

Superior sagittal sinus

Superior frontal gyrus

Cingulate gyrus

Corpus callosum

Lateral ventricle, frontal horn

Caudate nucleus

Internal capsule, corona radiata

Sylvian fissure

Fornix, along body of lateral ventricle

Lateral ventricle, atrium

Calcarine fissure

Superior sagittal sinus

Corpus callosum, splenium

Infratentorial structures

Straight sinus

Occipital lobe

Falx cerebri

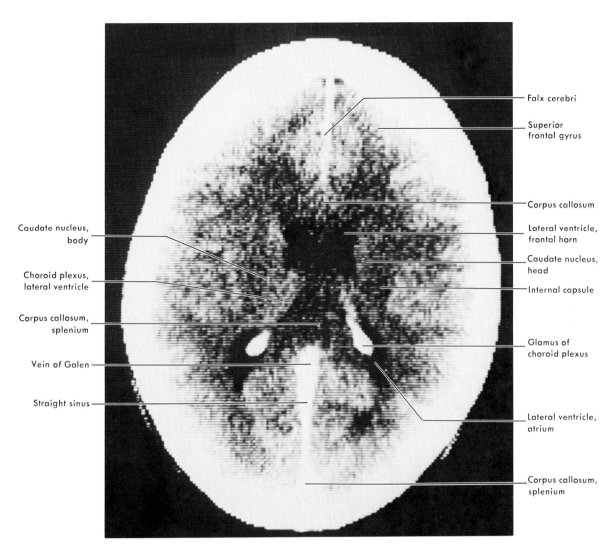

Falx cerebri

Superior
frontal gyrus

Corpus callosum

Lateral ventricle,
frontal horn

Caudate nucleus,
head

Internal capsule

Glomus of
choroid plexus

Lateral ventricle,
atrium

Corpus callosum,
splenium

Caudate nucleus,
body

Choroid plexus,
lateral ventricle

Corpus callosum,
splenium

Vein of Galen

Straight sinus

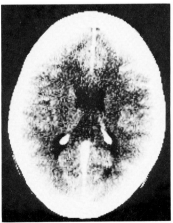

Computed tomography of the human body

Cingulate gyrus

Corpus callosum

Septum pellucidum

Anterior columns
of fornix

Septal vein

Anterior thalamus

Cistern of velum
interpositum

Choroid fissure

Vein of Galen

Lateral sinus

Caudate nucleus

Internal capsule, genu

Putamen

Insula

Sylvian fissure

Posterior thalamus

Fimbria of fornix

Hippocampus

Lateral ventricle,
temporal horn

Vermis of cerebellum

Tentorium of cerebellum

Straight sinus

Confluence of sinuses

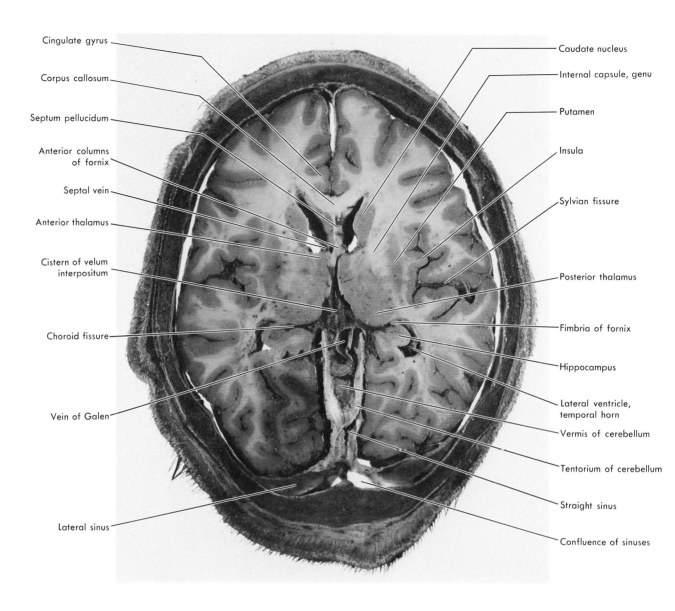

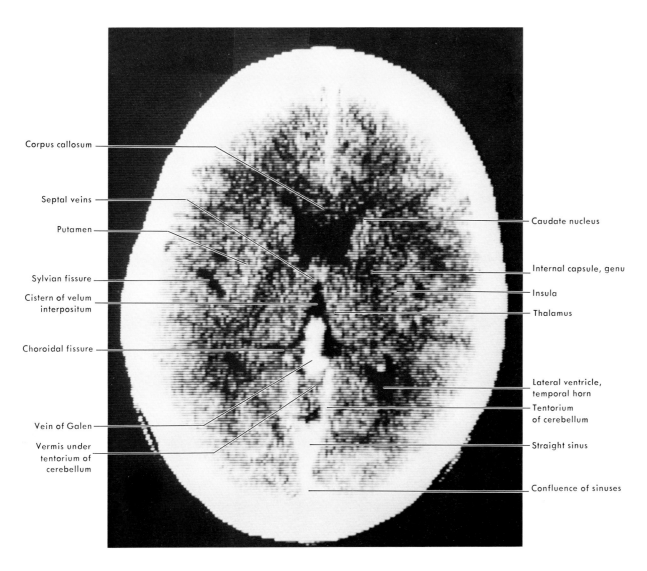

Corpus callosum

Septal veins

Putamen

Sylvian fissure

Cistern of velum interpositum

Choroidal fissure

Vein of Galen

Vermis under tentorium of cerebellum

Caudate nucleus

Internal capsule, genu

Insula

Thalamus

Lateral ventricle, temporal horn

Tentorium of cerebellum

Straight sinus

Confluence of sinuses

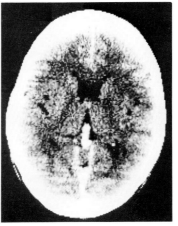

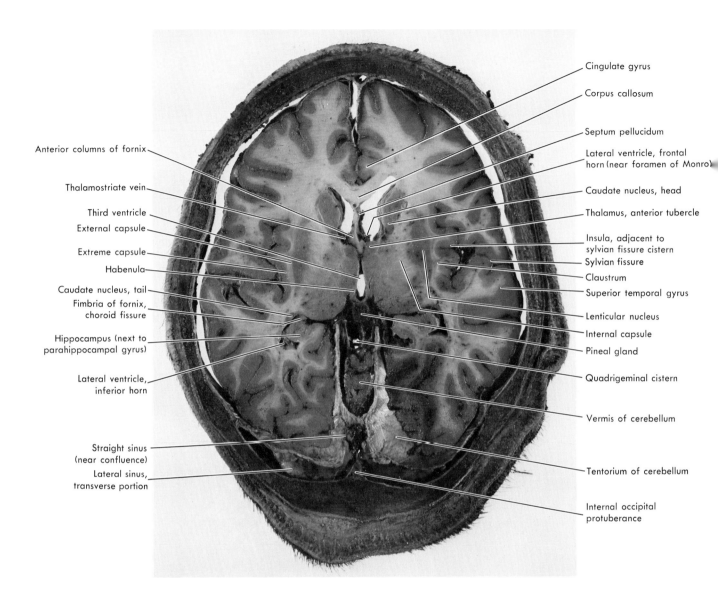

Cingulate gyrus

Corpus callosum

Septum pellucidum

Lateral ventricle, frontal horn (near foramen of Monro)

Caudate nucleus, head

Thalamus, anterior tubercle

Insula, adjacent to sylvian fissure cistern

Sylvian fissure

Claustrum

Superior temporal gyrus

Lenticular nucleus

Internal capsule

Pineal gland

Quadrigeminal cistern

Vermis of cerebellum

Tentorium of cerebellum

Internal occipital protuberance

Anterior columns of fornix

Thalamostriate vein

Third ventricle

External capsule

Extreme capsule

Habenula

Caudate nucleus, tail

Fimbria of fornix, choroid fissure

Hippocampus (next to parahippocampal gyrus)

Lateral ventricle, inferior horn

Straight sinus (near confluence)

Lateral sinus, transverse portion

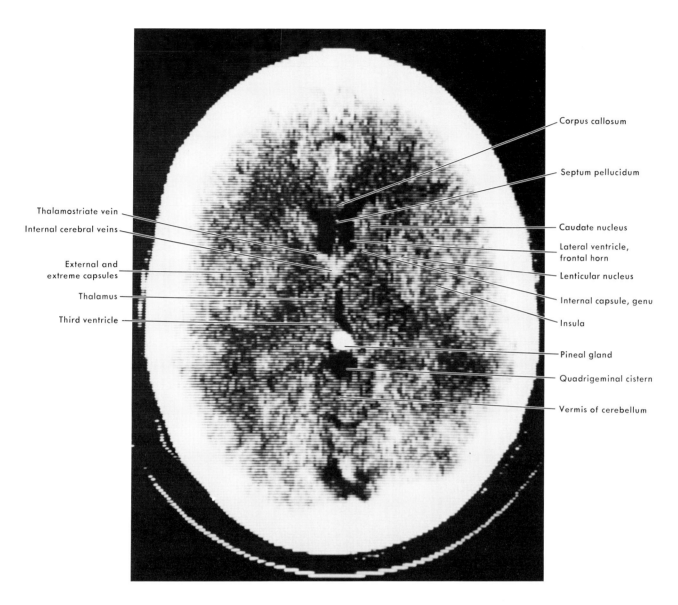

Corpus callosum

Septum pellucidum

Thalamostriate vein

Internal cerebral veins

Caudate nucleus

External and
extreme capsules

Lateral ventricle,
frontal horn

Thalamus

Lenticular nucleus

Internal capsule, genu

Third ventricle

Insula

Pineal gland

Quadrigeminal cistern

Vermis of cerebellum

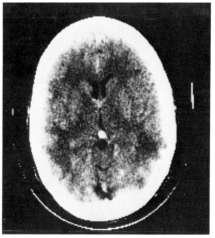

Computed tomography of the human body

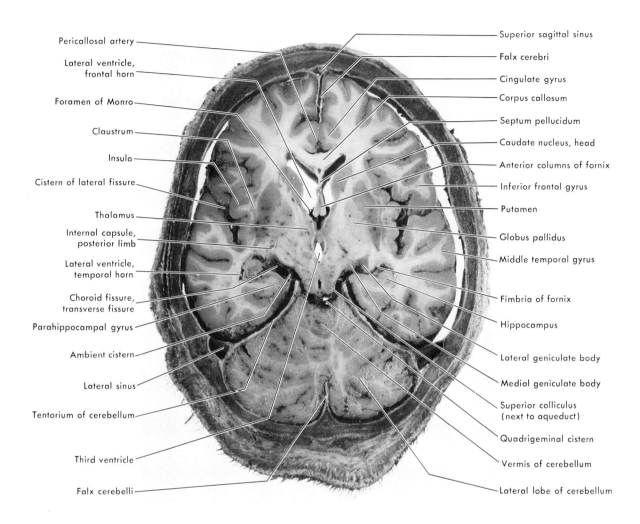

Pericallosal artery

Lateral ventricle, frontal horn

Foramen of Monro

Claustrum

Insula

Cistern of lateral fissure

Thalamus

Internal capsule, posterior limb

Lateral ventricle, temporal horn

Choroid fissure, transverse fissure

Parahippocampal gyrus

Ambient cistern

Lateral sinus

Tentorium of cerebellum

Third ventricle

Falx cerebelli

Superior sagittal sinus

Falx cerebri

Cingulate gyrus

Corpus callosum

Septum pellucidum

Caudate nucleus, head

Anterior columns of fornix

Inferior frontal gyrus

Putamen

Globus pallidus

Middle temporal gyrus

Fimbria of fornix

Hippocampus

Lateral geniculate body

Medial geniculate body

Superior colliculus (next to aqueduct)

Quadrigeminal cistern

Vermis of cerebellum

Lateral lobe of cerebellum

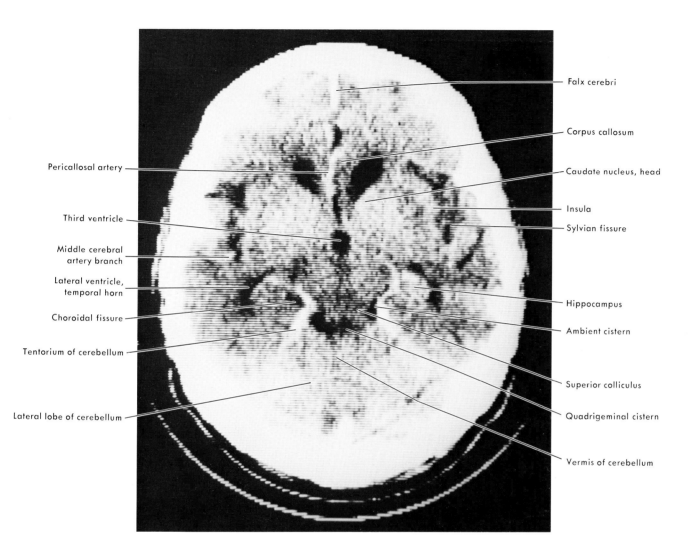

Falx cerebri

Corpus callosum

Caudate nucleus, head

Insula

Sylvian fissure

Pericallosal artery

Third ventricle

Middle cerebral
artery branch

Lateral ventricle,
temporal horn

Choroidal fissure

Tentorium of cerebellum

Lateral lobe of cerebellum

Hippocampus

Ambient cistern

Superior colliculus

Quadrigeminal cistern

Vermis of cerebellum

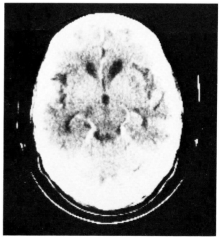

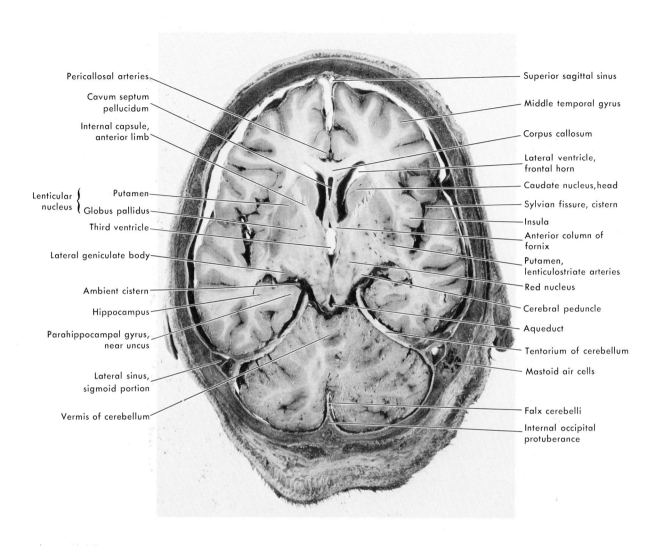

Pericallosal arteries

Cavum septum pellucidum

Internal capsule, anterior limb

Lenticular nucleus { Putamen

Globus pallidus

Third ventricle

Lateral geniculate body

Ambient cistern

Hippocampus

Parahippocampal gyrus, near uncus

Lateral sinus, sigmoid portion

Vermis of cerebellum

Superior sagittal sinus

Middle temporal gyrus

Corpus callosum

Lateral ventricle, frontal horn

Caudate nucleus, head

Sylvian fissure, cistern

Insula

Anterior column of fornix

Putamen, lenticulostriate arteries

Red nucleus

Cerebral peduncle

Aqueduct

Tentorium of cerebellum

Mastoid air cells

Falx cerebelli

Internal occipital protuberance

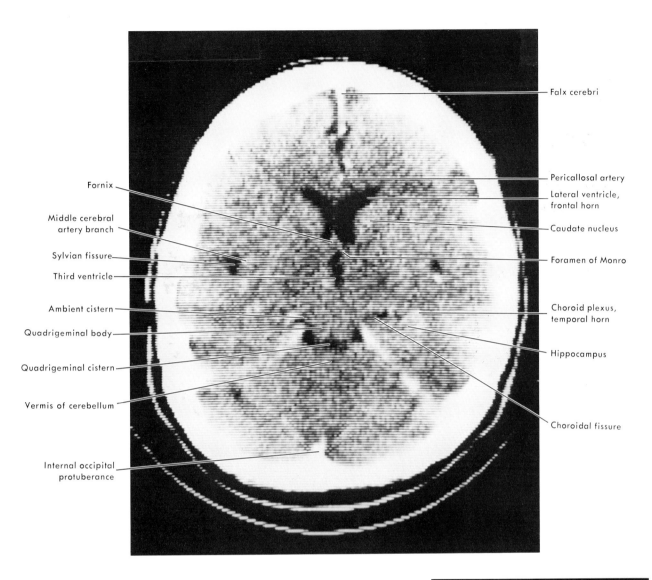

Falx cerebri

Pericallosal artery

Lateral ventricle, frontal horn

Caudate nucleus

Foramen of Monro

Choroid plexus, temporal horn

Hippocampus

Choroidal fissure

Fornix

Middle cerebral artery branch

Sylvian fissure

Third ventricle

Ambient cistern

Quadrigeminal body

Quadrigeminal cistern

Vermis of cerebellum

Internal occipital protuberance

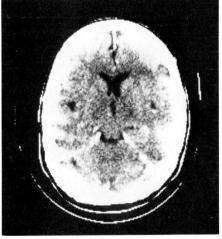

Computed tomography of the human body

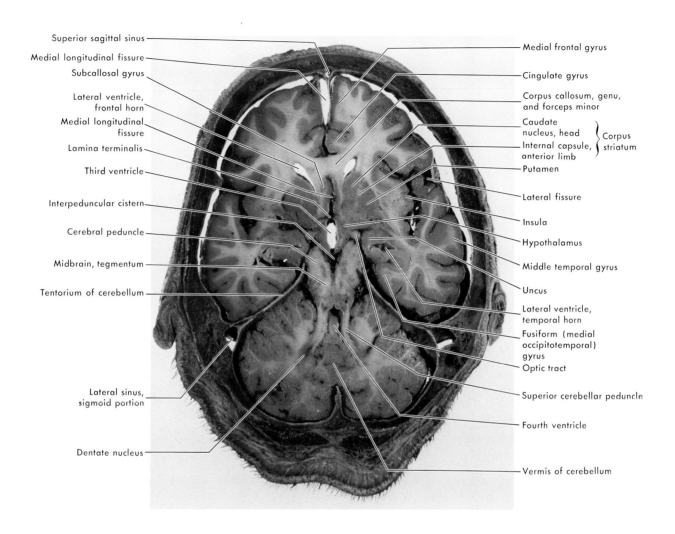

Superior sagittal sinus

Medial longitudinal fissure

Subcallosal gyrus

Lateral ventricle, frontal horn

Medial longitudinal fissure

Lamina terminalis

Third ventricle

Interpeduncular cistern

Cerebral peduncle

Midbrain, tegmentum

Tentorium of cerebellum

Lateral sinus, sigmoid portion

Dentate nucleus

Medial frontal gyrus

Cingulate gyrus

Corpus callosum, genu, and forceps minor

Caudate nucleus, head }
Internal capsule, anterior limb } Corpus striatum

Putamen

Lateral fissure

Insula

Hypothalamus

Middle temporal gyrus

Uncus

Lateral ventricle, temporal horn

Fusiform (medial occipitotemporal) gyrus

Optic tract

Superior cerebellar peduncle

Fourth ventricle

Vermis of cerebellum

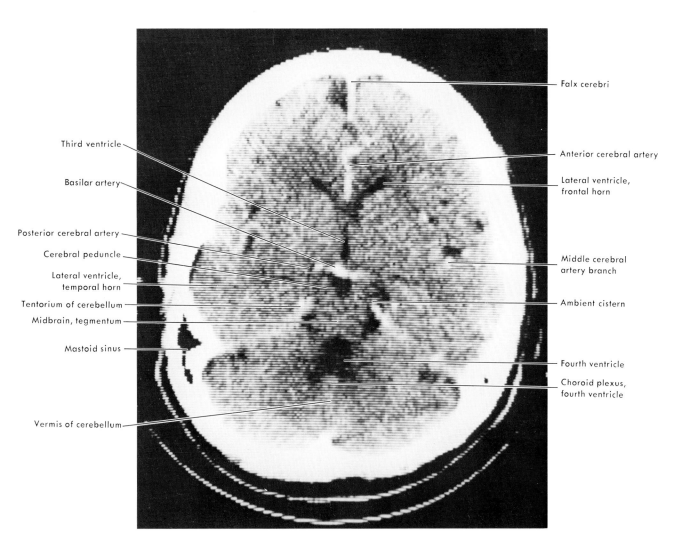

Falx cerebri

Third ventricle

Basilar artery

Posterior cerebral artery

Cerebral peduncle

Lateral ventricle, temporal horn

Tentorium of cerebellum

Midbrain, tegmentum

Mastoid sinus

Vermis of cerebellum

Anterior cerebral artery

Lateral ventricle, frontal horn

Middle cerebral artery branch

Ambient cistern

Fourth ventricle

Choroid plexus, fourth ventricle

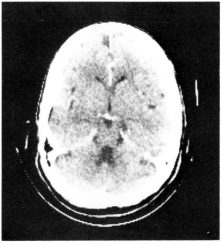

Computed tomography of the human body

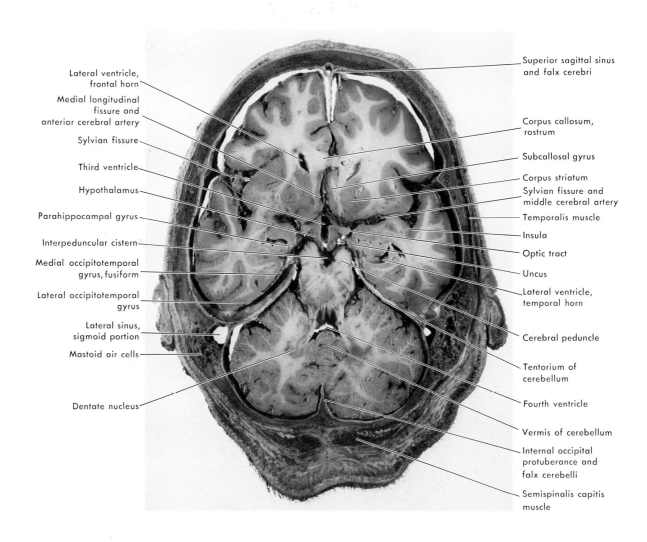

Lateral ventricle, frontal horn

Medial longitudinal fissure and anterior cerebral artery

Sylvian fissure

Third ventricle

Hypothalamus

Parahippocampal gyrus

Interpeduncular cistern

Medial occipitotemporal gyrus, fusiform

Lateral occipitotemporal gyrus

Lateral sinus, sigmoid portion

Mastoid air cells

Dentate nucleus

Superior sagittal sinus and falx cerebri

Corpus callosum, rostrum

Subcallosal gyrus

Corpus striatum

Sylvian fissure and middle cerebral artery

Temporalis muscle

Insula

Optic tract

Uncus

Lateral ventricle, temporal horn

Cerebral peduncle

Tentorium of cerebellum

Fourth ventricle

Vermis of cerebellum

Internal occipital protuberance and falx cerebelli

Semispinalis capitis muscle

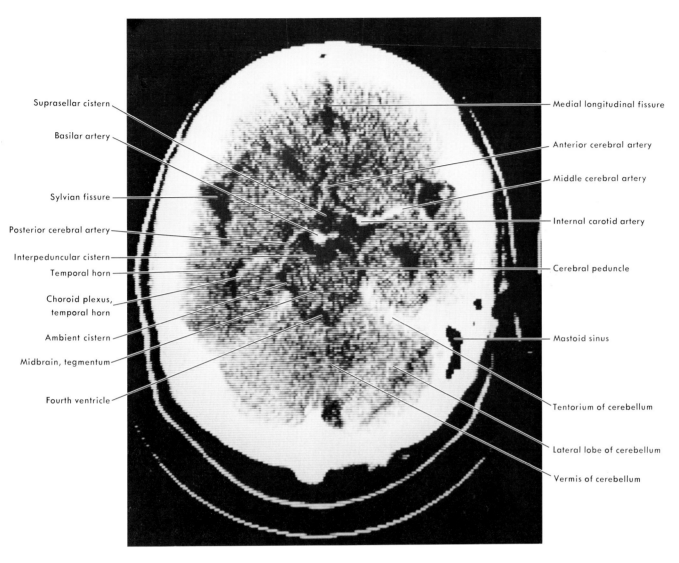

Suprasellar cistern

Basilar artery

Sylvian fissure

Posterior cerebral artery

Interpeduncular cistern

Temporal horn

Choroid plexus, temporal horn

Ambient cistern

Midbrain, tegmentum

Fourth ventricle

Medial longitudinal fissure

Anterior cerebral artery

Middle cerebral artery

Internal carotid artery

Cerebral peduncle

Mastoid sinus

Tentorium of cerebellum

Lateral lobe of cerebellum

Vermis of cerebellum

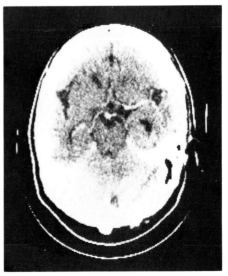

Computed tomography of the human body

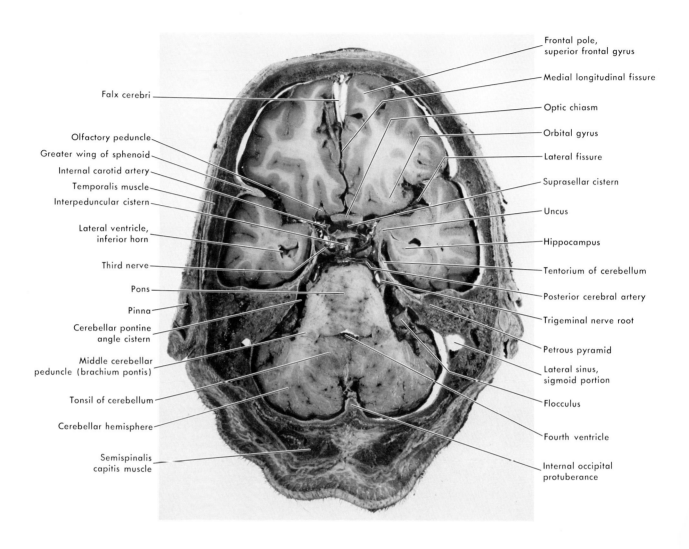

Falx cerebri

Olfactory peduncle
Greater wing of sphenoid
Internal carotid artery
Temporalis muscle
Interpeduncular cistern

Lateral ventricle,
inferior horn

Third nerve

Pons

Pinna

Cerebellar pontine
angle cistern

Middle cerebellar
peduncle (brachium pontis)

Tonsil of cerebellum

Cerebellar hemisphere

Semispinalis
capitis muscle

Frontal pole,
superior frontal gyrus

Medial longitudinal fissure

Optic chiasm

Orbital gyrus

Lateral fissure

Suprasellar cistern

Uncus

Hippocampus

Tentorium of cerebellum

Posterior cerebral artery

Trigeminal nerve root

Petrous pyramid

Lateral sinus,
sigmoid portion

Flocculus

Fourth ventricle

Internal occipital
protuberance

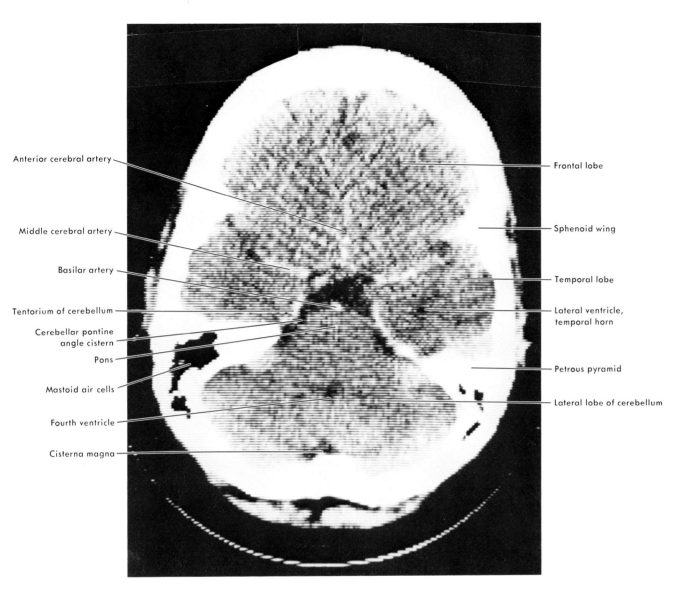

Anterior cerebral artery

Middle cerebral artery

Basilar artery

Tentorium of cerebellum

Cerebellar pontine
angle cistern

Pons

Mastoid air cells

Fourth ventricle

Cisterna magna

Frontal lobe

Sphenoid wing

Temporal lobe

Lateral ventricle,
temporal horn

Petrous pyramid

Lateral lobe of cerebellum

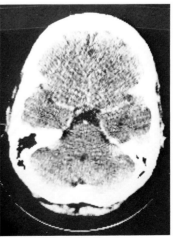

Computed tomography of the human body

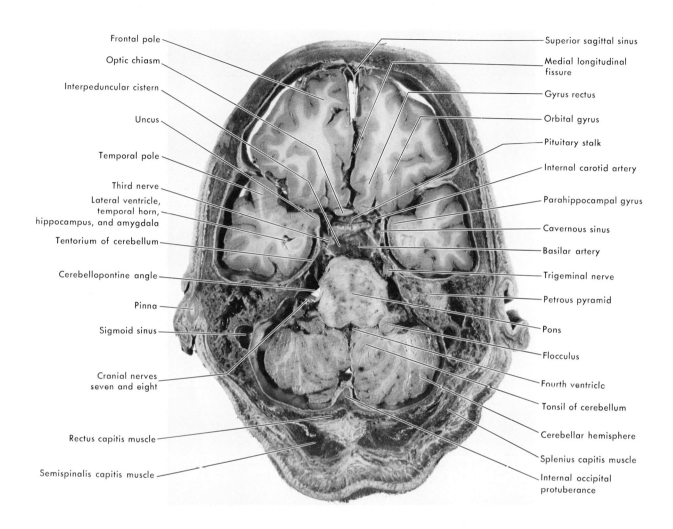

Frontal pole

Optic chiasm

Interpeduncular cistern

Uncus

Temporal pole

Third nerve

Lateral ventricle, temporal horn, hippocampus, and amygdala

Tentorium of cerebellum

Cerebellopontine angle

Pinna

Sigmoid sinus

Cranial nerves seven and eight

Rectus capitis muscle

Semispinalis capitis muscle

Superior sagittal sinus

Medial longitudinal fissure

Gyrus rectus

Orbital gyrus

Pituitary stalk

Internal carotid artery

Parahippocampal gyrus

Cavernous sinus

Basilar artery

Trigeminal nerve

Petrous pyramid

Pons

Flocculus

Fourth ventricle

Tonsil of cerebellum

Cerebellar hemisphere

Splenius capitis muscle

Internal occipital protuberance

32

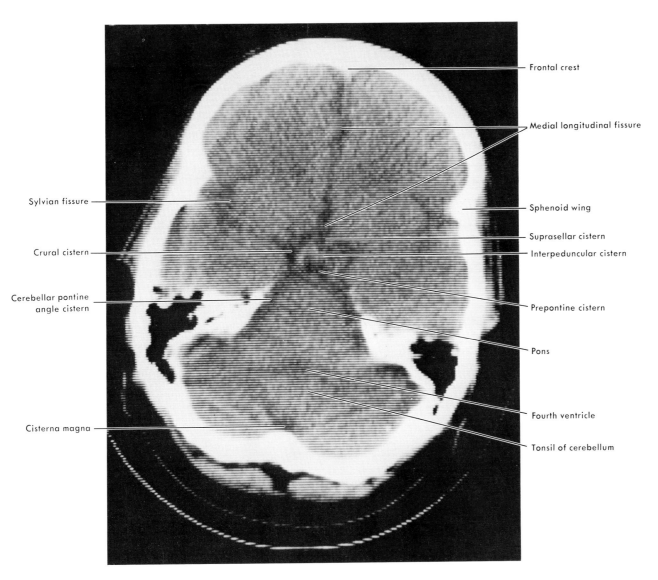

Frontal crest

Medial longitudinal fissure

Sylvian fissure

Sphenoid wing

Suprasellar cistern

Crural cistern

Interpeduncular cistern

Cerebellar pontine
angle cistern

Prepontine cistern

Pons

Fourth ventricle

Cisterna magna

Tonsil of cerebellum

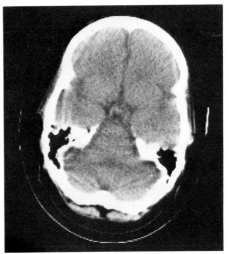

Computed tomography of the human body

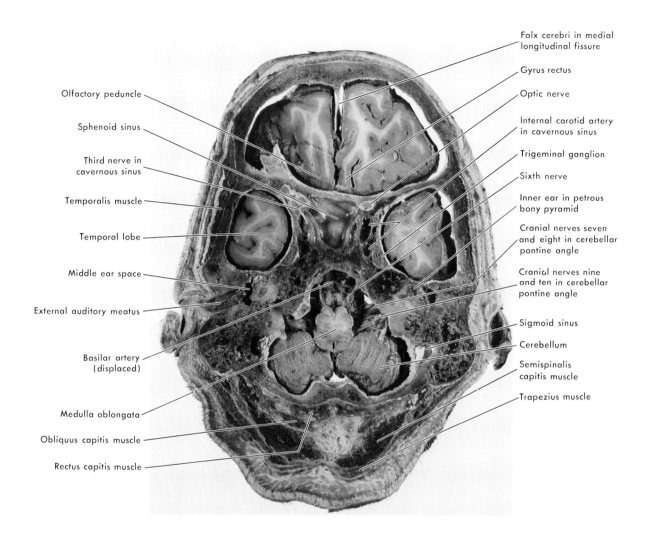

Olfactory peduncle

Sphenoid sinus

Third nerve in
cavernous sinus

Temporalis muscle

Temporal lobe

Middle ear space

External auditory meatus

Basilar artery
(displaced)

Medulla oblongata

Obliquus capitis muscle

Rectus capitis muscle

Falx cerebri in medial
longitudinal fissure

Gyrus rectus

Optic nerve

Internal carotid artery
in cavernous sinus

Trigeminal ganglion

Sixth nerve

Inner ear in petrous
bony pyramid

Cranial nerves seven
and eight in cerebellar
pontine angle

Cranial nerves nine
and ten in cerebellar
pontine angle

Sigmoid sinus

Cerebellum

Semispinalis
capitis muscle

Trapezius muscle

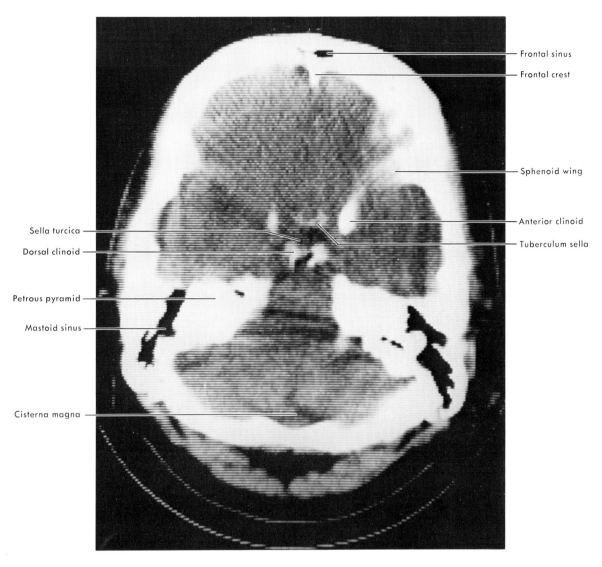

Frontal sinus

Frontal crest

Sphenoid wing

Anterior clinoid

Tuberculum sella

Sella turcica

Dorsal clinoid

Petrous pyramid

Mastoid sinus

Cisterna magna

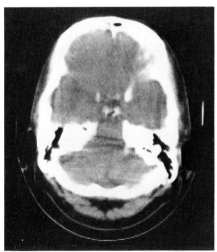

Computed tomography of the human body

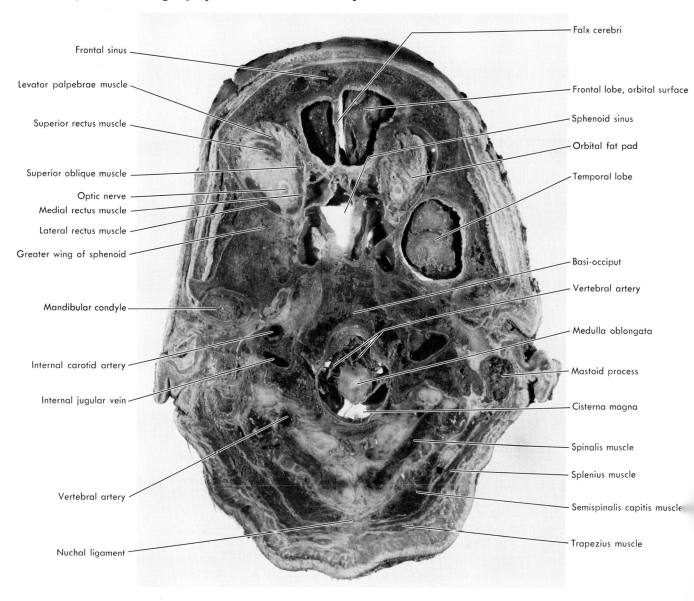

Frontal sinus

Levator palpebrae muscle

Superior rectus muscle

Superior oblique muscle

Optic nerve

Medial rectus muscle

Lateral rectus muscle

Greater wing of sphenoid

Mandibular condyle

Internal carotid artery

Internal jugular vein

Vertebral artery

Nuchal ligament

Falx cerebri

Frontal lobe, orbital surface

Sphenoid sinus

Orbital fat pad

Temporal lobe

Basi-occiput

Vertebral artery

Medulla oblongata

Mastoid process

Cisterna magna

Spinalis muscle

Splenius muscle

Semispinalis capitis muscle

Trapezius muscle

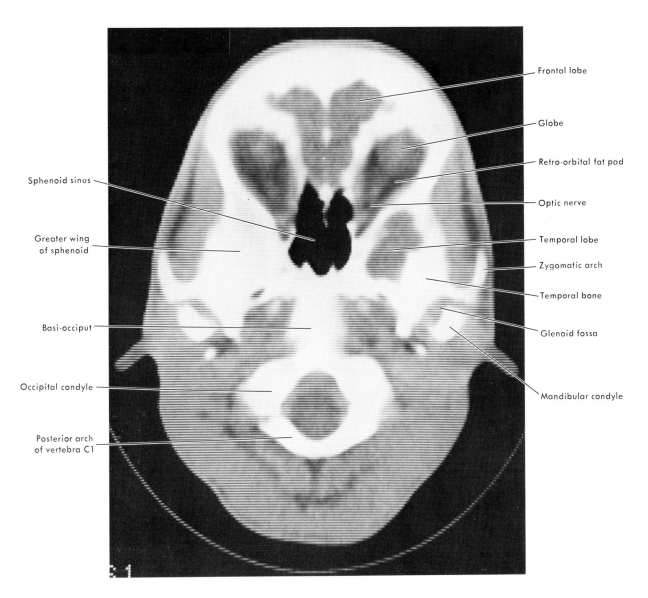

Frontal lobe

Globe

Retro-orbital fat pad

Optic nerve

Temporal lobe

Zygomatic arch

Temporal bone

Glenoid fossa

Mandibular condyle

Sphenoid sinus

Greater wing of sphenoid

Basi-occiput

Occipital condyle

Posterior arch of vertebra C1

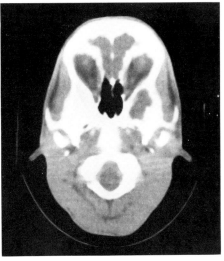

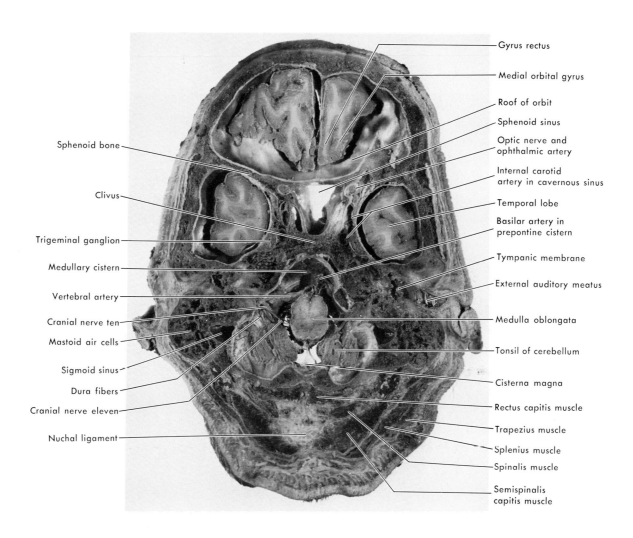

Gyrus rectus

Medial orbital gyrus

Roof of orbit

Sphenoid sinus

Optic nerve and ophthalmic artery

Internal carotid artery in cavernous sinus

Temporal lobe

Basilar artery in prepontine cistern

Tympanic membrane

External auditory meatus

Medulla oblongata

Tonsil of cerebellum

Cisterna magna

Rectus capitis muscle

Trapezius muscle

Splenius muscle

Spinalis muscle

Semispinalis capitis muscle

Sphenoid bone

Clivus

Trigeminal ganglion

Medullary cistern

Vertebral artery

Cranial nerve ten

Mastoid air cells

Sigmoid sinus

Dura fibers

Cranial nerve eleven

Nuchal ligament

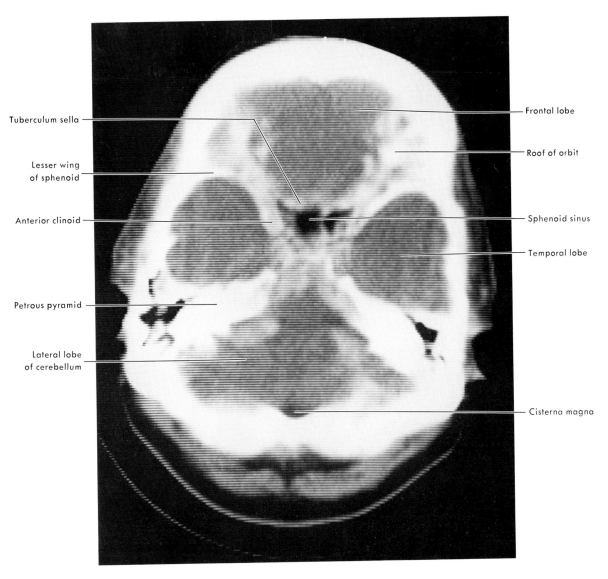

Tuberculum sella

Lesser wing
of sphenoid

Anterior clinoid

Petrous pyramid

Lateral lobe
of cerebellum

Frontal lobe

Roof of orbit

Sphenoid sinus

Temporal lobe

Cisterna magna

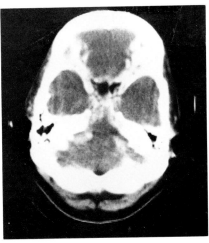

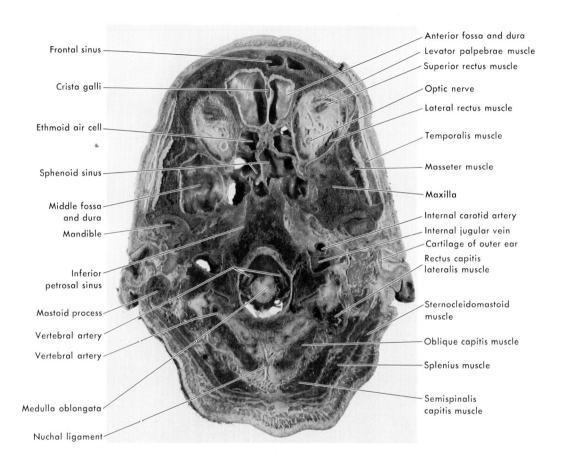

Frontal sinus

Crista galli

Ethmoid air cell

Sphenoid sinus

Middle fossa
and dura

Mandible

Inferior
petrosal sinus

Mastoid process

Vertebral artery

Vertebral artery

Medulla oblongata

Nuchal ligament

Anterior fossa and dura

Levator palpebrae muscle

Superior rectus muscle

Optic nerve

Lateral rectus muscle

Temporalis muscle

Masseter muscle

Maxilla

Internal carotid artery

Internal jugular vein

Cartilage of outer ear

Rectus capitis
lateralis muscle

Sternocleidomastoid
muscle

Oblique capitis muscle

Splenius muscle

Semispinalis
capitis muscle

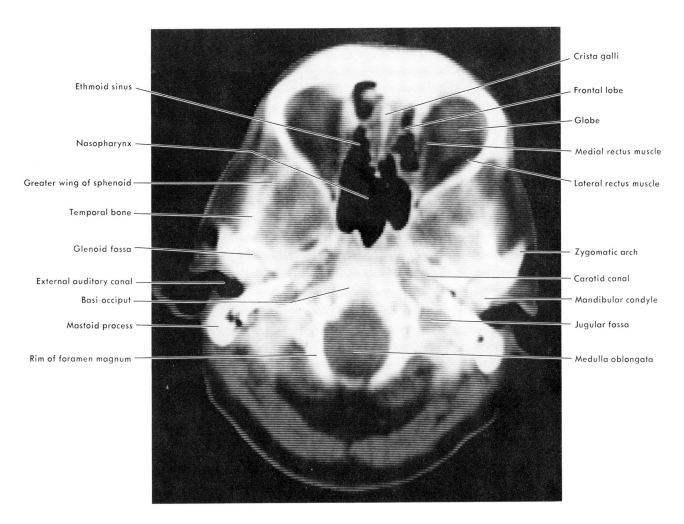

Ethmoid sinus

Nasopharynx

Greater wing of sphenoid

Temporal bone

Glenoid fossa

External auditory canal

Basi-occiput

Mastoid process

Rim of foramen magnum

Crista galli

Frontal lobe

Globe

Medial rectus muscle

Lateral rectus muscle

Zygomatic arch

Carotid canal

Mandibular condyle

Jugular fossa

Medulla oblongata

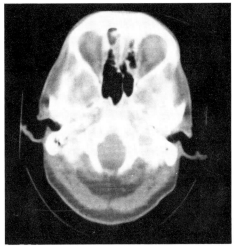

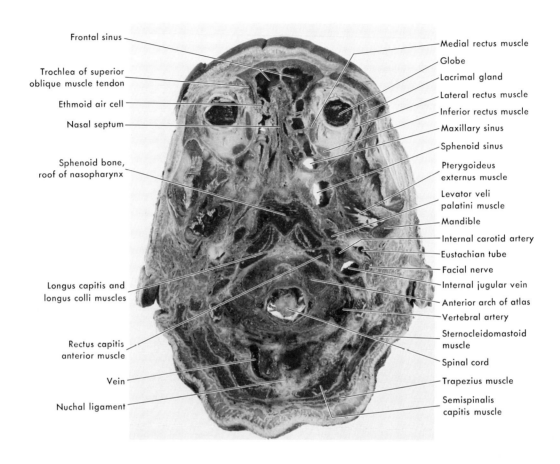

Frontal sinus

Trochlea of superior
oblique muscle tendon

Ethmoid air cell

Nasal septum

Sphenoid bone,
roof of nasopharynx

Longus capitis and
longus colli muscles

Rectus capitis
anterior muscle

Vein

Nuchal ligament

Medial rectus muscle

Globe

Lacrimal gland

Lateral rectus muscle

Inferior rectus muscle

Maxillary sinus

Sphenoid sinus

Pterygoideus
externus muscle

Levator veli
palatini muscle

Mandible

Internal carotid artery

Eustachian tube

Facial nerve

Internal jugular vein

Anterior arch of atlas

Vertebral artery

Sternocleidomastoid
muscle

Spinal cord

Trapezius muscle

Semispinalis
capitis muscle

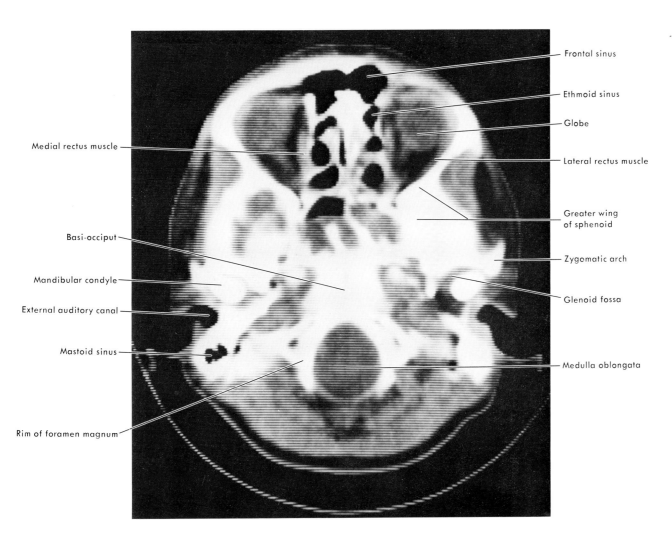

Frontal sinus

Ethmoid sinus

Globe

Medial rectus muscle

Lateral rectus muscle

Greater wing
of sphenoid

Basi-occiput

Zygomatic arch

Mandibular condyle

Glenoid fossa

External auditory canal

Mastoid sinus

Medulla oblongata

Rim of foramen magnum

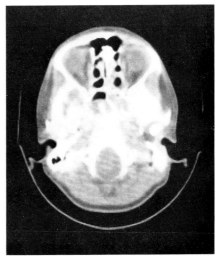

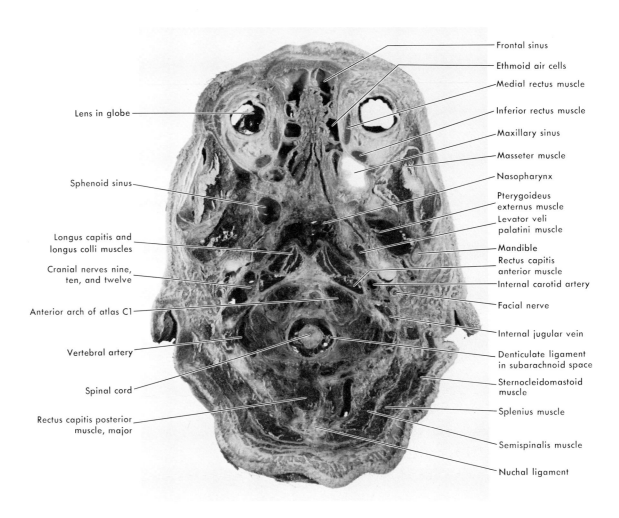

Lens in globe

Sphenoid sinus

Longus capitis and
longus colli muscles

Cranial nerves nine,
ten, and twelve

Anterior arch of atlas C1

Vertebral artery

Spinal cord

Rectus capitis posterior
muscle, major

Frontal sinus

Ethmoid air cells

Medial rectus muscle

Inferior rectus muscle

Maxillary sinus

Masseter muscle

Nasopharynx

Pterygoideus
externus muscle

Levator veli
palatini muscle

Mandible

Rectus capitis
anterior muscle

Internal carotid artery

Facial nerve

Internal jugular vein

Denticulate ligament
in subarachnoid space

Sternocleidomastoid
muscle

Splenius muscle

Semispinalis muscle

Nuchal ligament

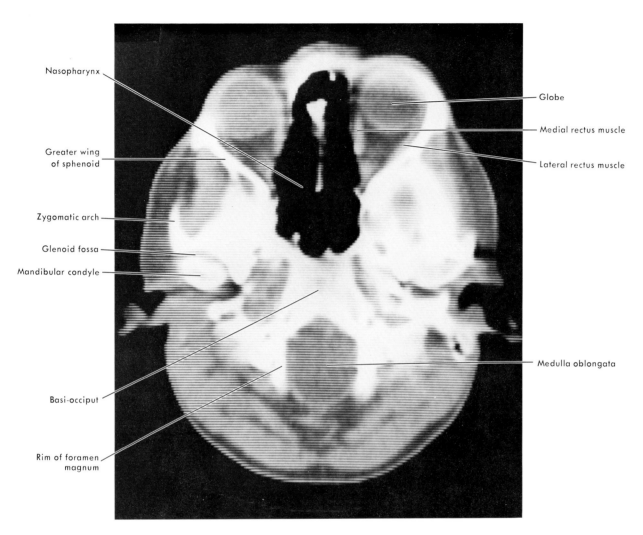

Nasopharynx

Greater wing of sphenoid

Zygomatic arch

Glenoid fossa

Mandibular condyle

Basi-occiput

Rim of foramen magnum

Globe

Medial rectus muscle

Lateral rectus muscle

Medulla oblongata

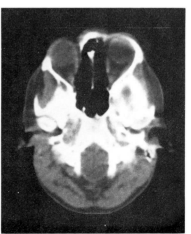

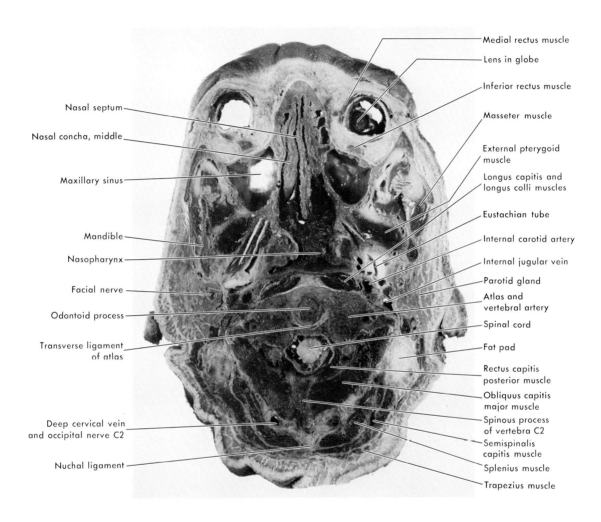

Medial rectus muscle

Lens in globe

Inferior rectus muscle

Masseter muscle

External pterygoid muscle

Longus capitis and longus colli muscles

Eustachian tube

Internal carotid artery

Internal jugular vein

Parotid gland

Atlas and vertebral artery

Spinal cord

Fat pad

Rectus capitis posterior muscle

Obliquus capitis major muscle

Spinous process of vertebra C2

Semispinalis capitis muscle

Splenius muscle

Trapezius muscle

Nasal septum

Nasal concha, middle

Maxillary sinus

Mandible

Nasopharynx

Facial nerve

Odontoid process

Transverse ligament of atlas

Deep cervical vein and occipital nerve C2

Nuchal ligament

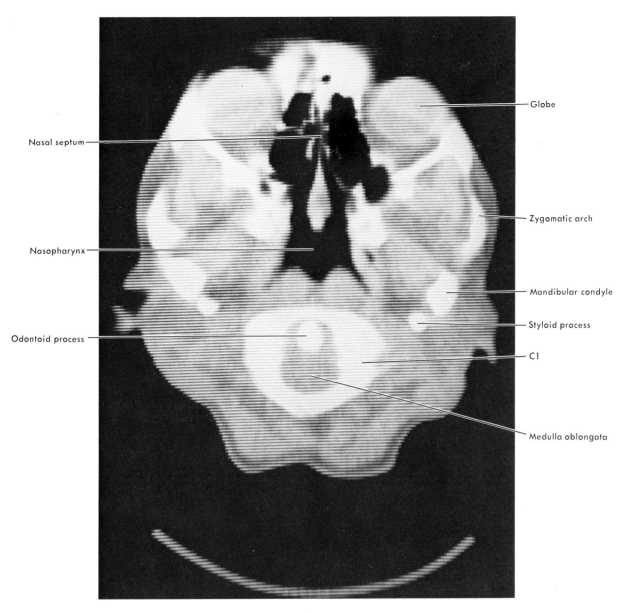

Globe

Nasal septum

Zygomatic arch

Nasopharynx

Mandibular condyle

Styloid process

Odontoid process

C1

Medulla oblongata

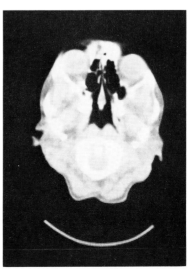

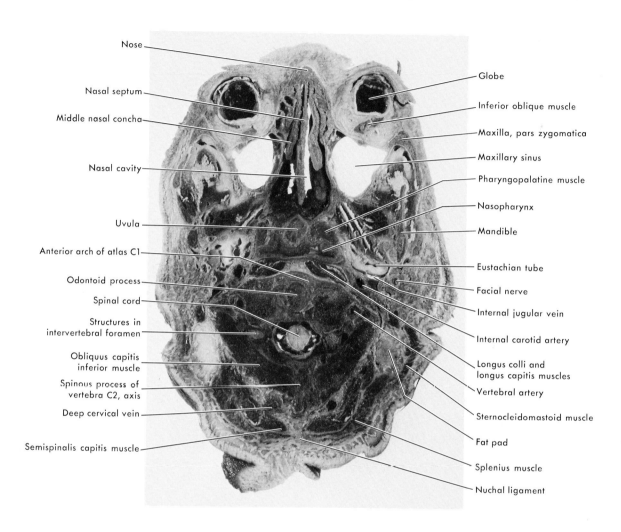

Nose

Nasal septum

Middle nasal concha

Nasal cavity

Uvula

Anterior arch of atlas C1

Odontoid process

Spinal cord

Structures in
intervertebral foramen

Obliquus capitis
inferior muscle

Spinous process of
vertebra C2, axis

Deep cervical vein

Semispinalis capitis muscle

Globe

Inferior oblique muscle

Maxilla, pars zygomatica

Maxillary sinus

Pharyngopalatine muscle

Nasopharynx

Mandible

Eustachian tube

Facial nerve

Internal jugular vein

Internal carotid artery

Longus colli and
longus capitis muscles

Vertebral artery

Sternocleidomastoid muscle

Fat pad

Splenius muscle

Nuchal ligament

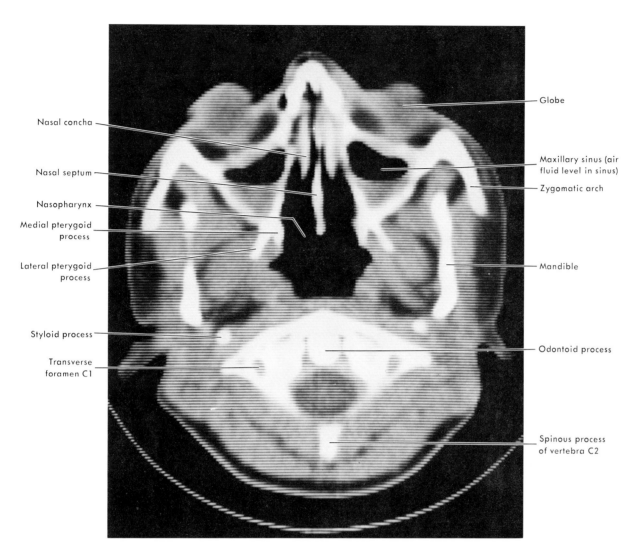

Nasal concha

Nasal septum

Nasopharynx

Medial pterygoid
process

Lateral pterygoid
process

Styloid process

Transverse
foramen C1

Globe

Maxillary sinus (air
fluid level in sinus)

Zygomatic arch

Mandible

Odontoid process

Spinous process
of vertebra C2

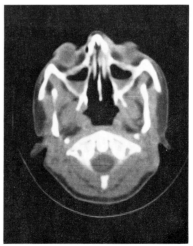

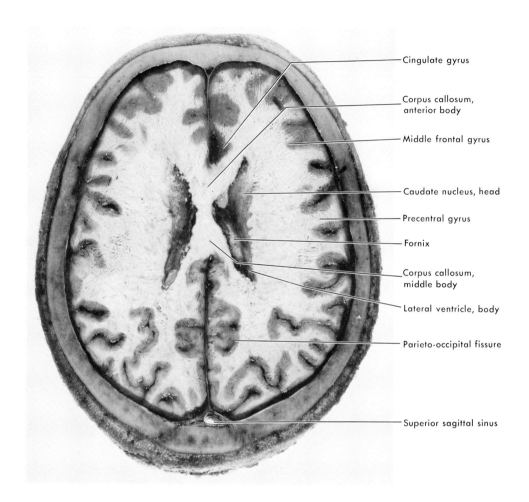

Cingulate gyrus

Corpus callosum, anterior body

Middle frontal gyrus

Caudate nucleus, head

Precentral gyrus

Fornix

Corpus callosum, middle body

Lateral ventricle, body

Parieto-occipital fissure

Superior sagittal sinus

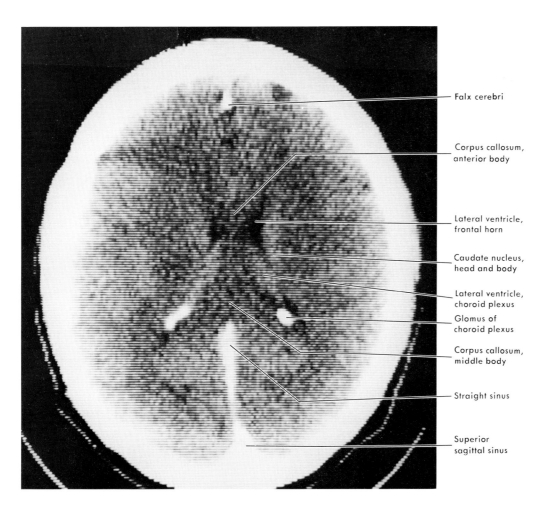

Falx cerebri

Corpus callosum, anterior body

Lateral ventricle, frontal horn

Caudate nucleus, head and body

Lateral ventricle, choroid plexus

Glomus of choroid plexus

Corpus callosum, middle body

Straight sinus

Superior sagittal sinus

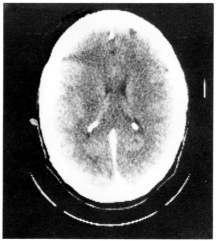

Computed tomography of the human body

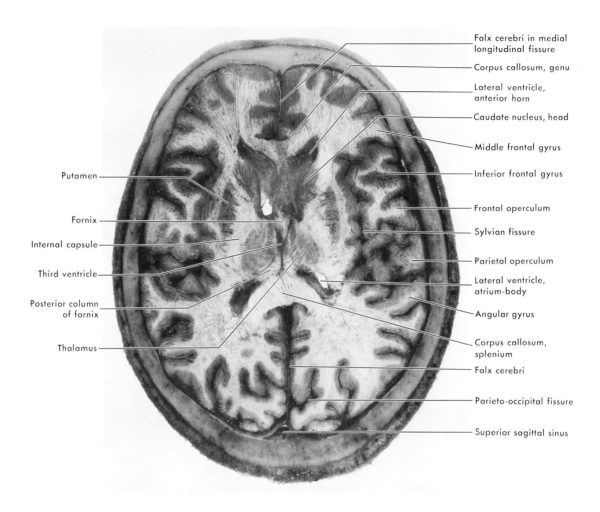

Falx cerebri in medial longitudinal fissure

Corpus callosum, genu

Lateral ventricle, anterior horn

Caudate nucleus, head

Middle frontal gyrus

Inferior frontal gyrus

Frontal operculum

Sylvian fissure

Parietal operculum

Lateral ventricle, atrium-body

Angular gyrus

Corpus callosum, splenium

Falx cerebri

Parieto-occipital fissure

Superior sagittal sinus

Putamen

Fornix

Internal capsule

Third ventricle

Posterior column of fornix

Thalamus

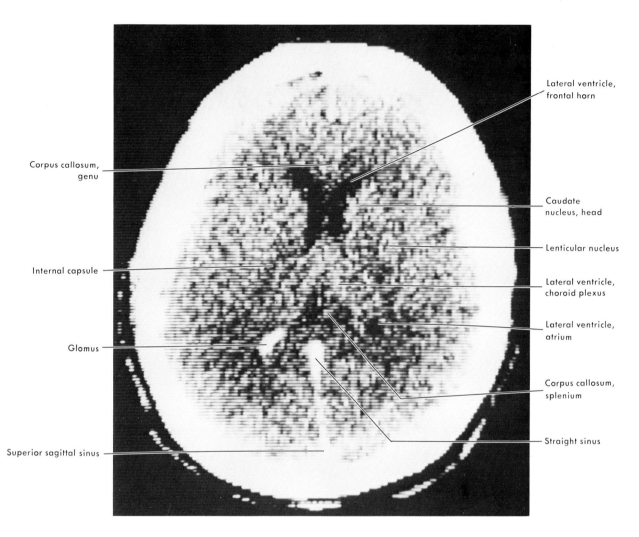

Lateral ventricle,
frontal horn

Corpus callosum,
genu

Caudate
nucleus, head

Lenticular nucleus

Internal capsule

Lateral ventricle,
choroid plexus

Lateral ventricle,
atrium

Glomus

Corpus callosum,
splenium

Superior sagittal sinus

Straight sinus

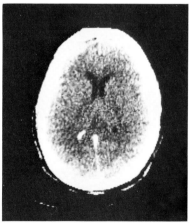

Computed tomography of the human body

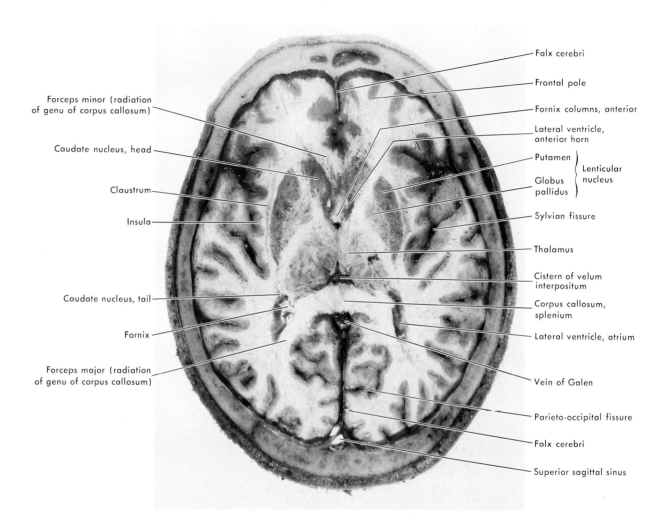

Falx cerebri

Frontal pole

Fornix columns, anterior

Lateral ventricle, anterior horn

Putamen

Globus pallidus — Lenticular nucleus

Sylvian fissure

Thalamus

Cistern of velum interpositum

Corpus callosum, splenium

Lateral ventricle, atrium

Vein of Galen

Parieto-occipital fissure

Falx cerebri

Superior sagittal sinus

Forceps minor (radiation of genu of corpus callosum)

Caudate nucleus, head

Claustrum

Insula

Caudate nucleus, tail

Fornix

Forceps major (radiation of genu of corpus callosum)

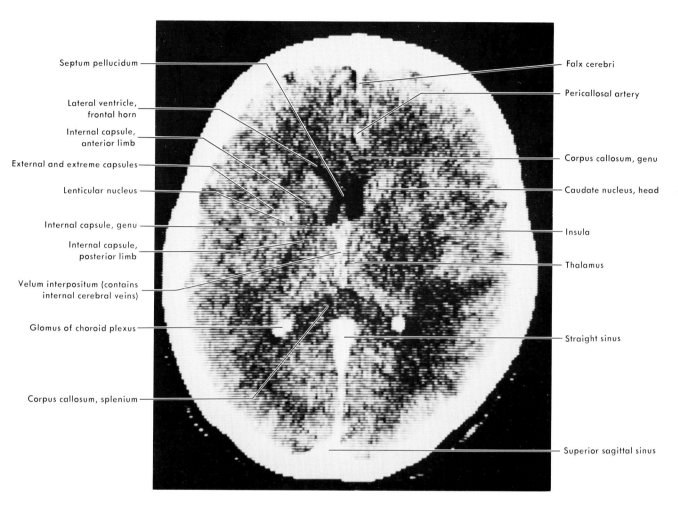

Septum pellucidum

Lateral ventricle,
frontal horn

Internal capsule,
anterior limb

External and extreme capsules

Lenticular nucleus

Internal capsule, genu

Internal capsule,
posterior limb

Velum interpositum (contains
internal cerebral veins)

Glomus of choroid plexus

Corpus callosum, splenium

Falx cerebri

Pericallosal artery

Corpus callosum, genu

Caudate nucleus, head

Insula

Thalamus

Straight sinus

Superior sagittal sinus

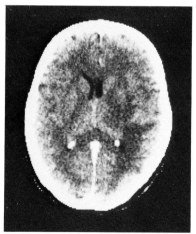

Computed tomography of the human body

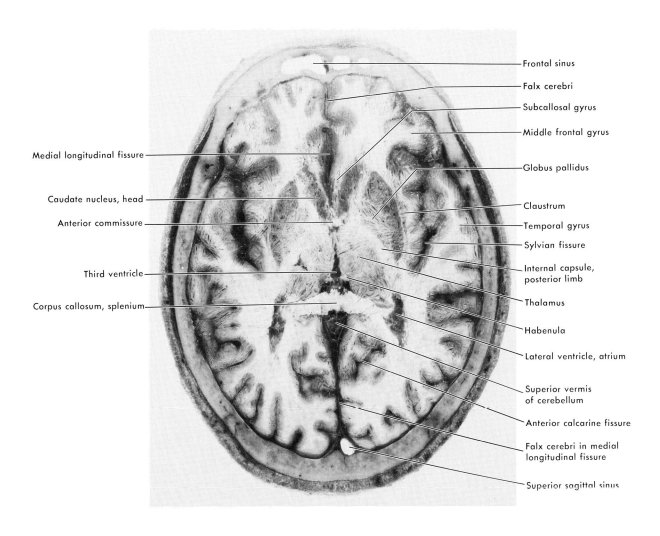

Frontal sinus

Falx cerebri

Subcallosal gyrus

Middle frontal gyrus

Medial longitudinal fissure

Globus pallidus

Caudate nucleus, head

Claustrum

Anterior commissure

Temporal gyrus

Sylvian fissure

Third ventricle

Internal capsule, posterior limb

Corpus callosum, splenium

Thalamus

Habenula

Lateral ventricle, atrium

Superior vermis of cerebellum

Anterior calcarine fissure

Falx cerebri in medial longitudinal fissure

Superior sagittal sinus

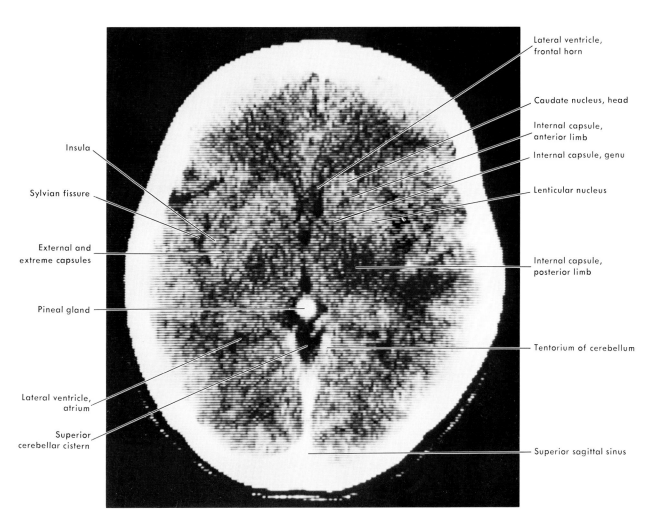

Insula

Sylvian fissure

External and
extreme capsules

Pineal gland

Lateral ventricle,
atrium

Superior
cerebellar cistern

Lateral ventricle,
frontal horn

Caudate nucleus, head

Internal capsule,
anterior limb

Internal capsule, genu

Lenticular nucleus

Internal capsule,
posterior limb

Tentorium of cerebellum

Superior sagittal sinus

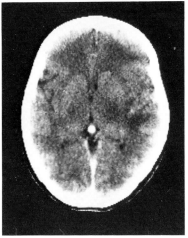

Computed tomography of the human body

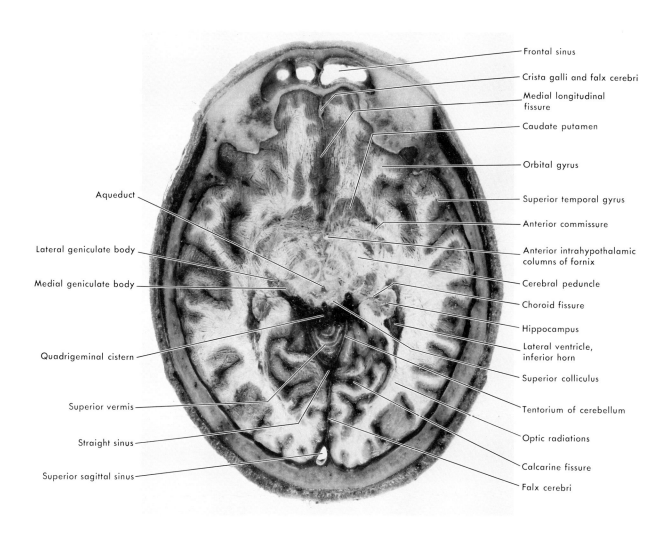

Frontal sinus

Crista galli and falx cerebri

Medial longitudinal fissure

Caudate putamen

Orbital gyrus

Superior temporal gyrus

Anterior commissure

Anterior intrahypothalamic columns of fornix

Cerebral peduncle

Choroid fissure

Hippocampus

Lateral ventricle, inferior horn

Superior colliculus

Tentorium of cerebellum

Optic radiations

Calcarine fissure

Falx cerebri

Aqueduct

Lateral geniculate body

Medial geniculate body

Quadrigeminal cistern

Superior vermis

Straight sinus

Superior sagittal sinus

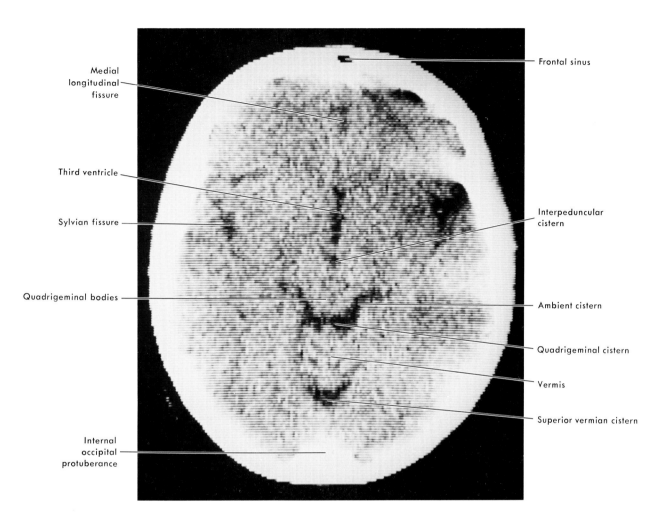

Medial longitudinal fissure

Frontal sinus

Third ventricle

Sylvian fissure

Interpeduncular cistern

Quadrigeminal bodies

Ambient cistern

Quadrigeminal cistern

Vermis

Superior vermian cistern

Internal occipital protuberance

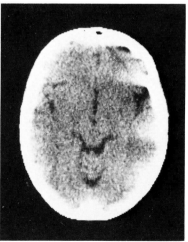

Computed tomography of the human body

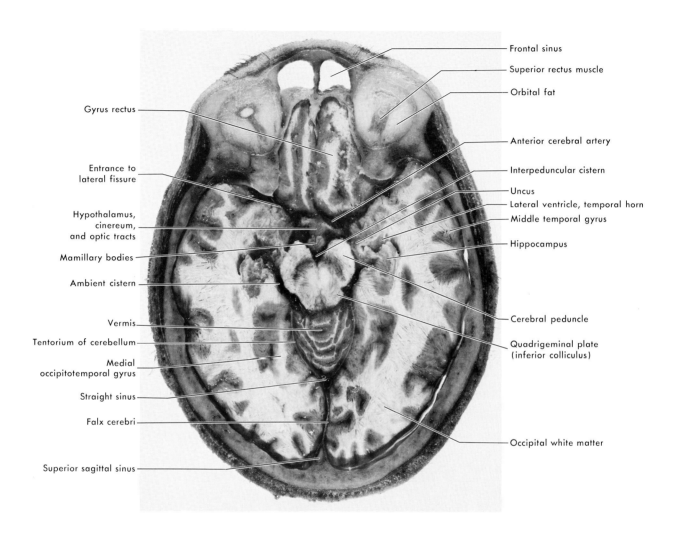

Gyrus rectus

Entrance to
lateral fissure

Hypothalamus,
cinereum,
and optic tracts

Mamillary bodies

Ambient cistern

Vermis

Tentorium of cerebellum

Medial
occipitotemporal gyrus

Straight sinus

Falx cerebri

Superior sagittal sinus

Frontal sinus

Superior rectus muscle

Orbital fat

Anterior cerebral artery

Interpeduncular cistern

Uncus

Lateral ventricle, temporal horn

Middle temporal gyrus

Hippocampus

Cerebral peduncle

Quadrigeminal plate
(inferior colliculus)

Occipital white matter

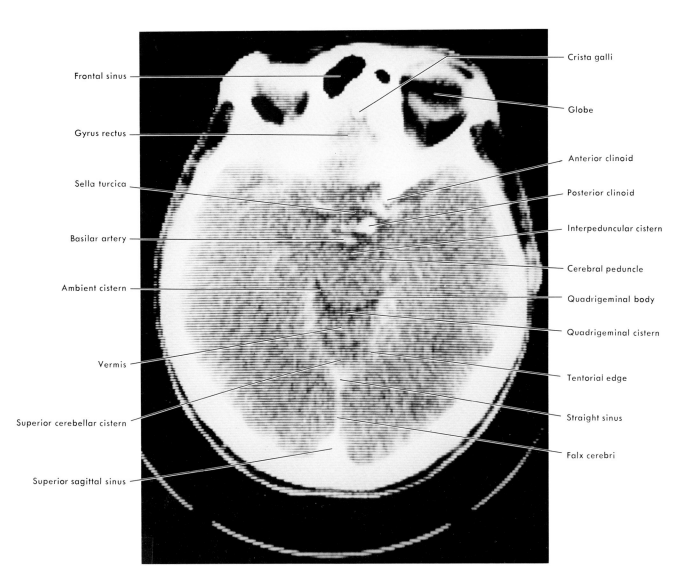

Frontal sinus

Gyrus rectus

Sella turcica

Basilar artery

Ambient cistern

Vermis

Superior cerebellar cistern

Superior sagittal sinus

Crista galli

Globe

Anterior clinoid

Posterior clinoid

Interpeduncular cistern

Cerebral peduncle

Quadrigeminal body

Quadrigeminal cistern

Tentorial edge

Straight sinus

Falx cerebri

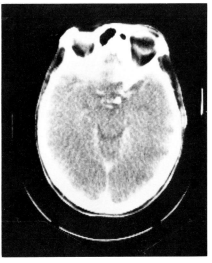

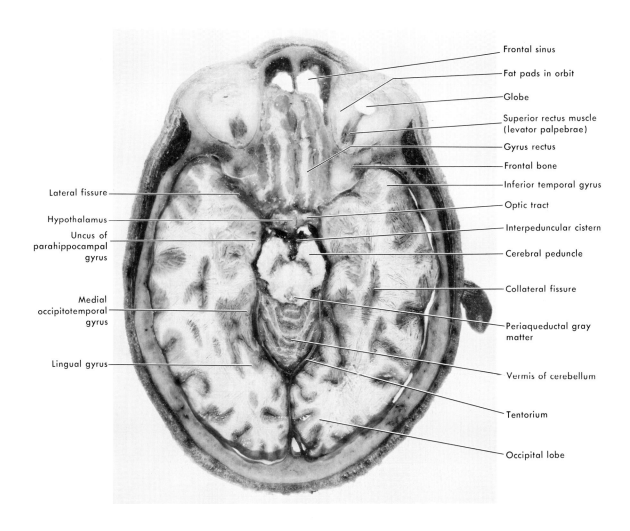

Frontal sinus

Fat pads in orbit

Globe

Superior rectus muscle (levator palpebrae)

Gyrus rectus

Frontal bone

Inferior temporal gyrus

Optic tract

Interpeduncular cistern

Cerebral peduncle

Collateral fissure

Periaqueductal gray matter

Vermis of cerebellum

Tentorium

Occipital lobe

Lateral fissure

Hypothalamus

Uncus of parahippocampal gyrus

Medial occipitotemporal gyrus

Lingual gyrus

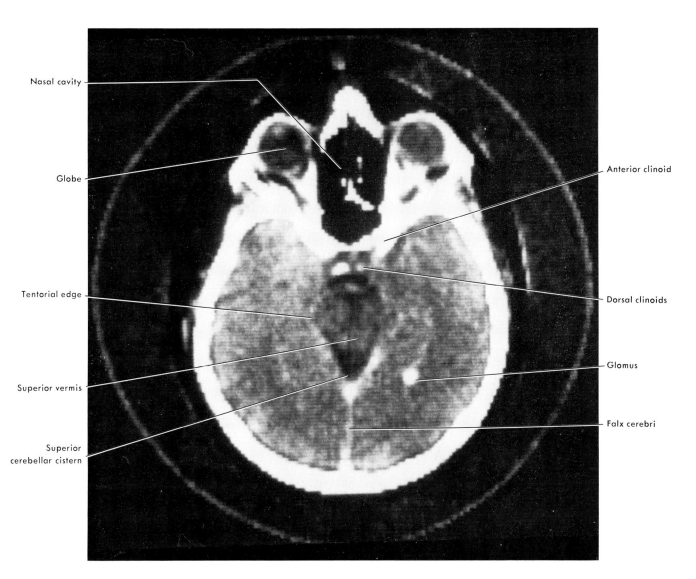

Nasal cavity

Globe

Tentorial edge

Superior vermis

Superior
cerebellar cistern

Anterior clinoid

Dorsal clinoids

Glomus

Falx cerebri

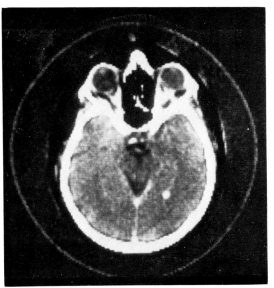

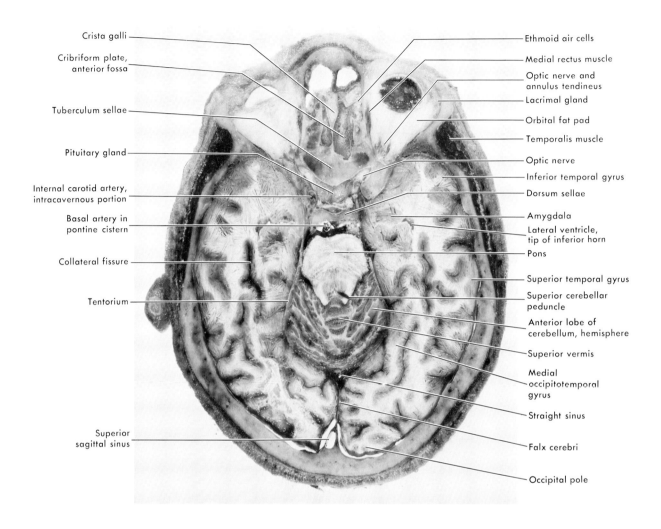

Crista galli

Cribriform plate, anterior fossa

Tuberculum sellae

Pituitary gland

Internal carotid artery, intracavernous portion

Basal artery in pontine cistern

Collateral fissure

Tentorium

Superior sagittal sinus

Ethmoid air cells

Medial rectus muscle

Optic nerve and annulus tendineus

Lacrimal gland

Orbital fat pad

Temporalis muscle

Optic nerve

Inferior temporal gyrus

Dorsum sellae

Amygdala

Lateral ventricle, tip of inferior horn

Pons

Superior temporal gyrus

Superior cerebellar peduncle

Anterior lobe of cerebellum, hemisphere

Superior vermis

Medial occipitotemporal gyrus

Straight sinus

Falx cerebri

Occipital pole

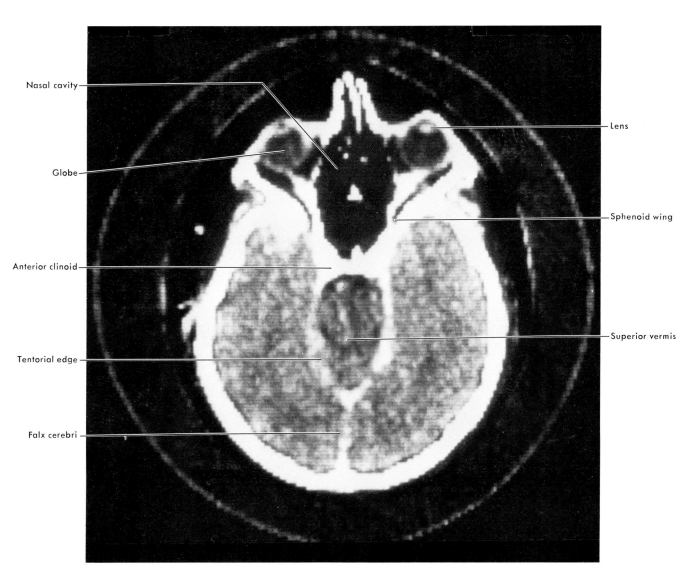

Nasal cavity

Lens

Globe

Anterior clinoid

Sphenoid wing

Tentorial edge

Superior vermis

Falx cerebri

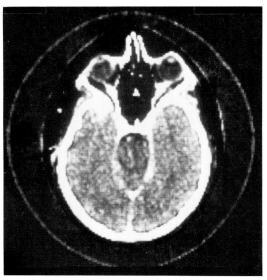

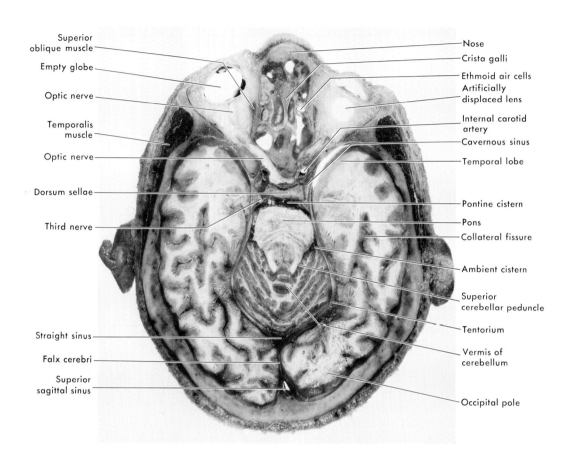

Superior oblique muscle

Empty globe

Optic nerve

Temporalis muscle

Optic nerve

Dorsum sellae

Third nerve

Straight sinus

Falx cerebri

Superior sagittal sinus

Nose

Crista galli

Ethmoid air cells

Artificially displaced lens

Internal carotid artery

Cavernous sinus

Temporal lobe

Pontine cistern

Pons

Collateral fissure

Ambient cistern

Superior cerebellar peduncle

Tentorium

Vermis of cerebellum

Occipital pole

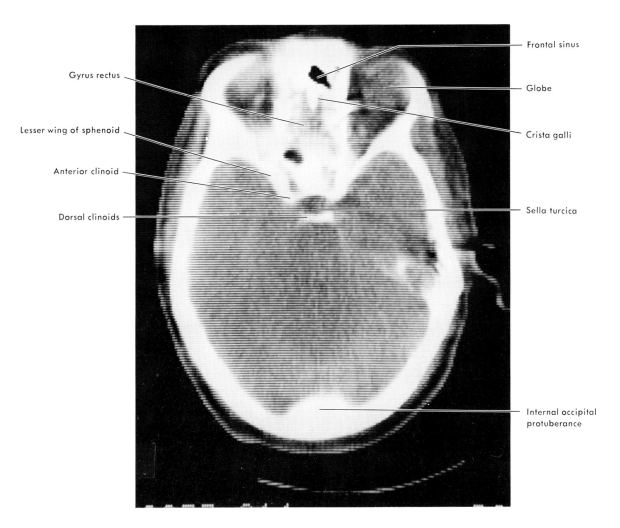

Gyrus rectus

Lesser wing of sphenoid

Anterior clinoid

Dorsal clinoids

Frontal sinus

Globe

Crista galli

Sella turcica

Internal occipital protuberance

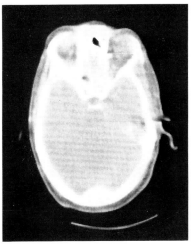

Computed tomography of the human body

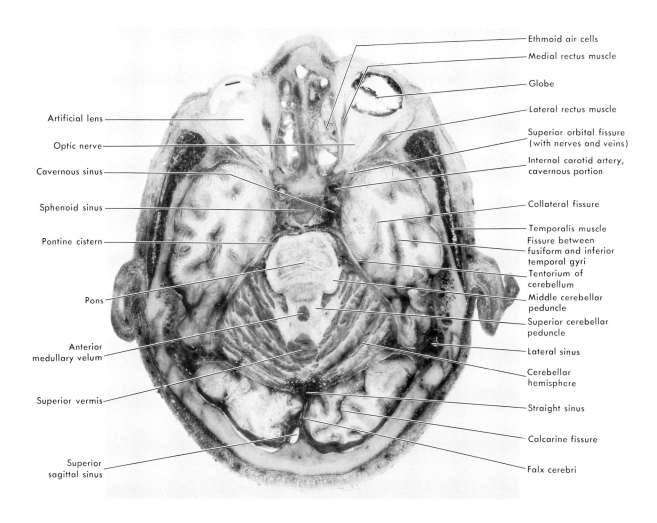

Ethmoid air cells

Medial rectus muscle

Globe

Lateral rectus muscle

Superior orbital fissure (with nerves and veins)

Internal carotid artery, cavernous portion

Collateral fissure

Temporalis muscle

Fissure between fusiform and inferior temporal gyri

Tentorium of cerebellum

Middle cerebellar peduncle

Superior cerebellar peduncle

Lateral sinus

Cerebellar hemisphere

Straight sinus

Calcarine fissure

Falx cerebri

Artificial lens

Optic nerve

Cavernous sinus

Sphenoid sinus

Pontine cistern

Pons

Anterior medullary velum

Superior vermis

Superior sagittal sinus

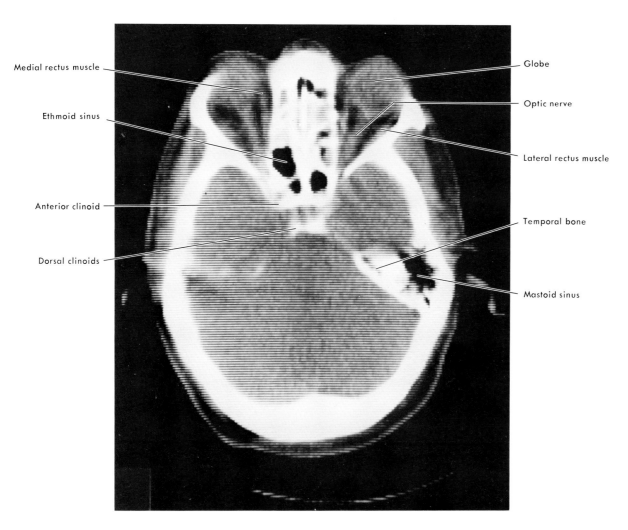

Medial rectus muscle

Ethmoid sinus

Anterior clinoid

Dorsal clinoids

Globe

Optic nerve

Lateral rectus muscle

Temporal bone

Mastoid sinus

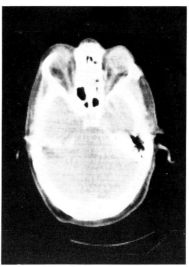

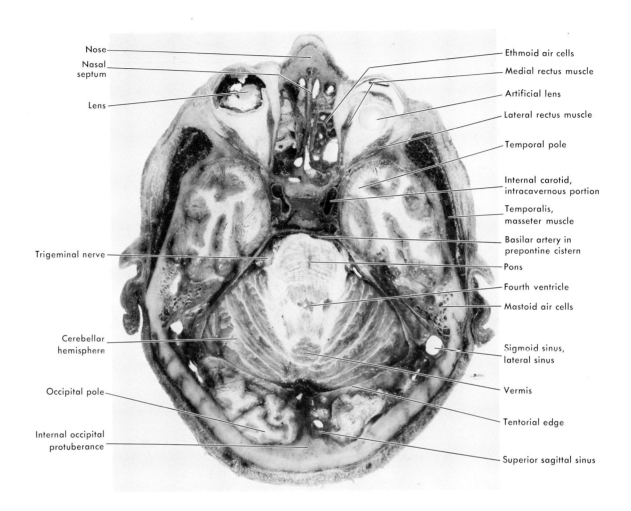

Nose

Nasal septum

Lens

Trigeminal nerve

Cerebellar hemisphere

Occipital pole

Internal occipital protuberance

Ethmoid air cells

Medial rectus muscle

Artificial lens

Lateral rectus muscle

Temporal pole

Internal carotid, intracavernous portion

Temporalis, masseter muscle

Basilar artery in prepontine cistern

Pons

Fourth ventricle

Mastoid air cells

Sigmoid sinus, lateral sinus

Vermis

Tentorial edge

Superior sagittal sinus

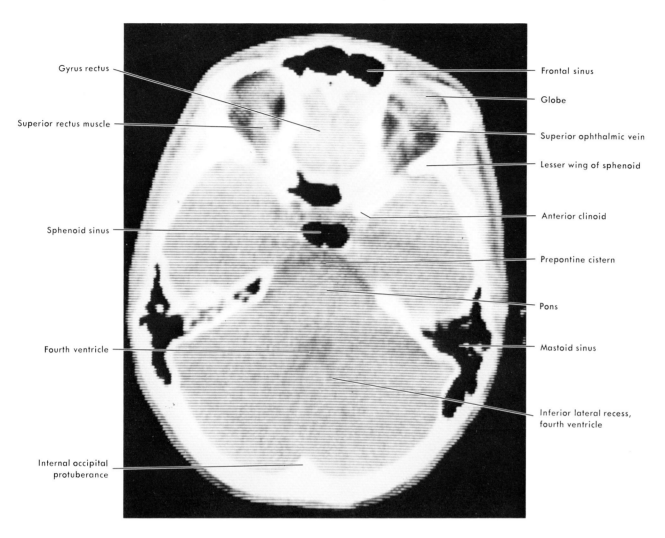

Gyrus rectus

Superior rectus muscle

Sphenoid sinus

Fourth ventricle

Internal occipital
protuberance

Frontal sinus

Globe

Superior ophthalmic vein

Lesser wing of sphenoid

Anterior clinoid

Prepontine cistern

Pons

Mastoid sinus

Inferior lateral recess,
fourth ventricle

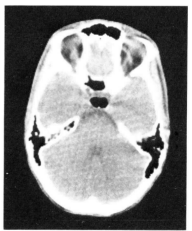

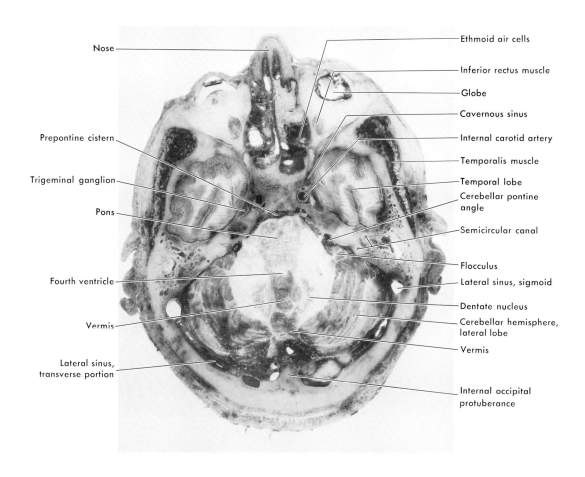

Nose

Prepontine cistern

Trigeminal ganglion

Pons

Fourth ventricle

Vermis

Lateral sinus, transverse portion

Ethmoid air cells

Inferior rectus muscle

Globe

Cavernous sinus

Internal carotid artery

Temporalis muscle

Temporal lobe

Cerebellar pontine angle

Semicircular canal

Flocculus

Lateral sinus, sigmoid

Dentate nucleus

Cerebellar hemisphere, lateral lobe

Vermis

Internal occipital protuberance

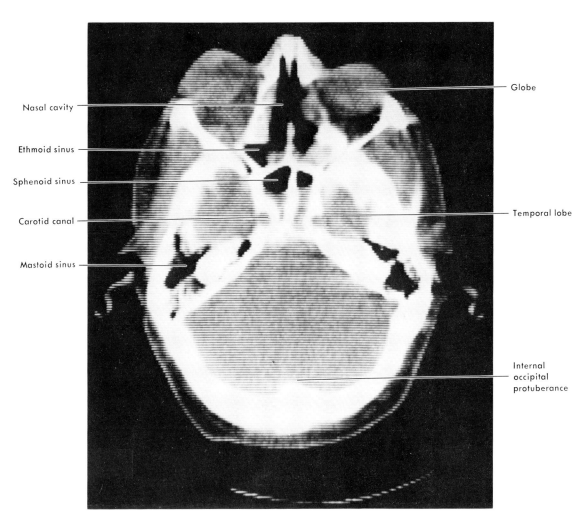

Nasal cavity

Ethmoid sinus

Sphenoid sinus

Carotid canal

Mastoid sinus

Globe

Temporal lobe

Internal
occipital
protuberance

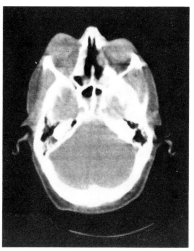

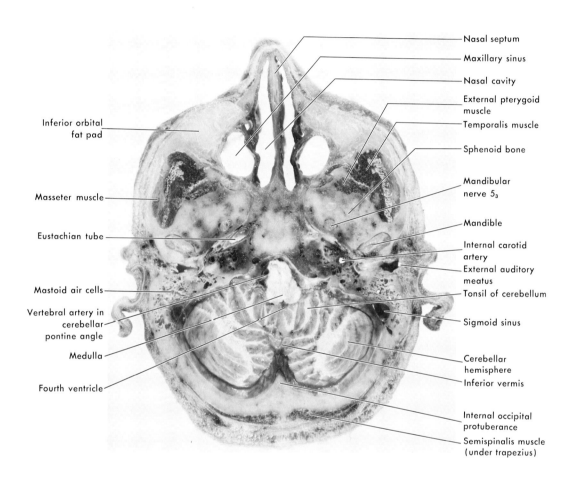

Nasal septum

Maxillary sinus

Nasal cavity

External pterygoid muscle

Temporalis muscle

Sphenoid bone

Mandibular nerve 5_3

Mandible

Internal carotid artery

External auditory meatus

Tonsil of cerebellum

Sigmoid sinus

Cerebellar hemisphere

Inferior vermis

Internal occipital protuberance

Semispinalis muscle (under trapezius)

Inferior orbital fat pad

Masseter muscle

Eustachian tube

Mastoid air cells

Vertebral artery in cerebellar pontine angle

Medulla

Fourth ventricle

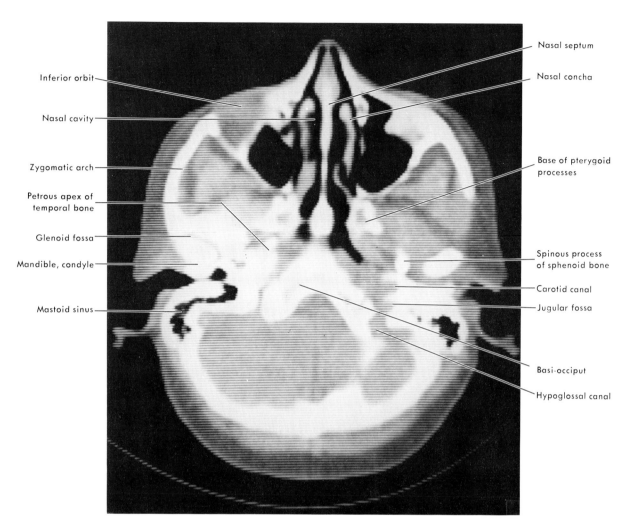

Inferior orbit

Nasal cavity

Zygomatic arch

Petrous apex of temporal bone

Glenoid fossa

Mandible, condyle

Mastoid sinus

Nasal septum

Nasal concha

Base of pterygoid processes

Spinous process of sphenoid bone

Carotid canal

Jugular fossa

Basi-occiput

Hypoglossal canal

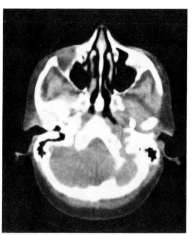

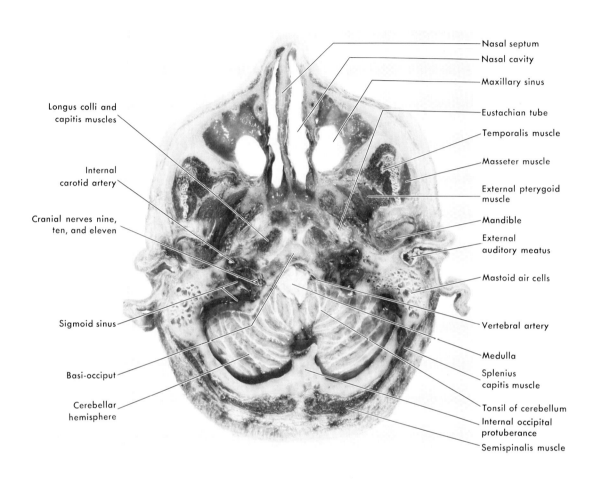

Nasal septum

Nasal cavity

Maxillary sinus

Longus colli and
capitis muscles

Eustachian tube

Temporalis muscle

Masseter muscle

Internal
carotid artery

External pterygoid
muscle

Cranial nerves nine,
ten, and eleven

Mandible

External
auditory meatus

Mastoid air cells

Sigmoid sinus

Vertebral artery

Medulla

Basi-occiput

Splenius
capitis muscle

Cerebellar
hemisphere

Tonsil of cerebellum

Internal occipital
protuberance

Semispinalis muscle

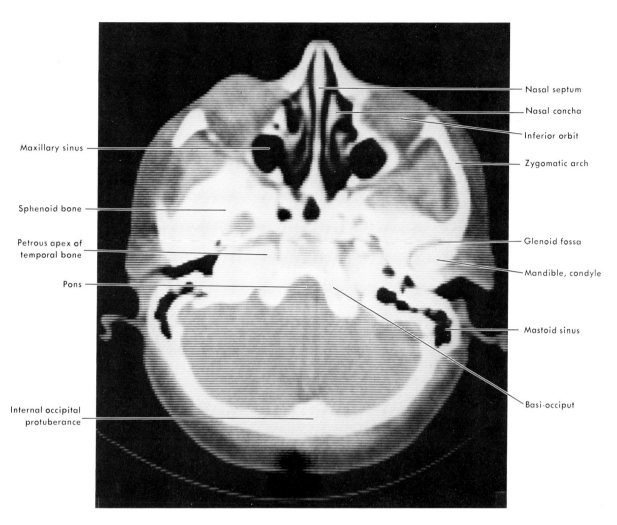

Maxillary sinus

Sphenoid bone

Petrous apex of
temporal bone

Pons

Internal occipital
protuberance

Nasal septum

Nasal concha

Inferior orbit

Zygomatic arch

Glenoid fossa

Mandible, condyle

Mastoid sinus

Basi-occiput

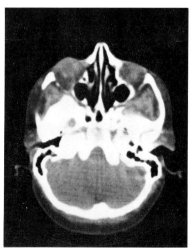

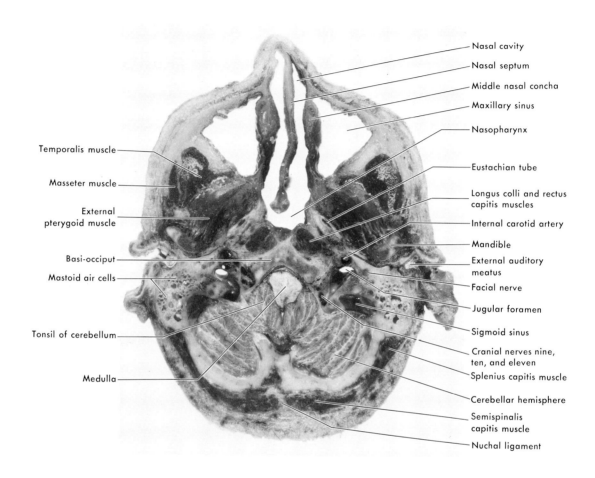

Nasal cavity

Nasal septum

Middle nasal concha

Maxillary sinus

Nasopharynx

Temporalis muscle

Eustachian tube

Masseter muscle

Longus colli and rectus capitis muscles

External pterygoid muscle

Internal carotid artery

Mandible

Basi-occiput

External auditory meatus

Mastoid air cells

Facial nerve

Jugular foramen

Tonsil of cerebellum

Sigmoid sinus

Cranial nerves nine, ten, and eleven

Medulla

Splenius capitis muscle

Cerebellar hemisphere

Semispinalis capitis muscle

Nuchal ligament

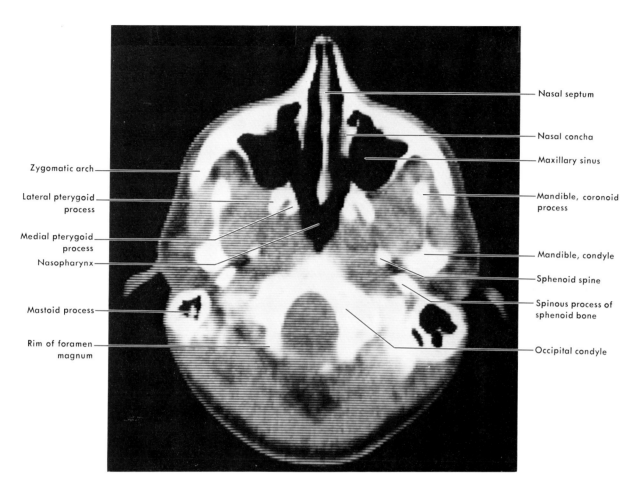

Nasal septum

Nasal concha

Maxillary sinus

Zygomatic arch

Lateral pterygoid process

Mandible, coronoid process

Medial pterygoid process

Nasopharynx

Mandible, condyle

Sphenoid spine

Spinous process of sphenoid bone

Mastoid process

Rim of foramen magnum

Occipital condyle

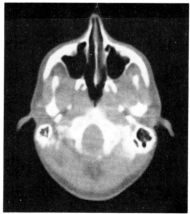

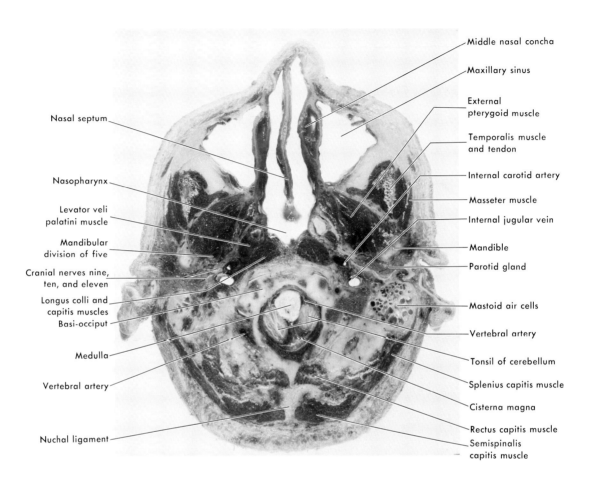

Nasal septum

Nasopharynx

Levator veli
palatini muscle

Mandibular
division of five

Cranial nerves nine,
ten, and eleven

Longus colli and
capitis muscles

Basi-occiput

Medulla

Vertebral artery

Nuchal ligament

Middle nasal concha

Maxillary sinus

External
pterygoid muscle

Temporalis muscle
and tendon

Internal carotid artery

Masseter muscle

Internal jugular vein

Mandible

Parotid gland

Mastoid air cells

Vertebral artery

Tonsil of cerebellum

Splenius capitis muscle

Cisterna magna

Rectus capitis muscle

Semispinalis
capitis muscle

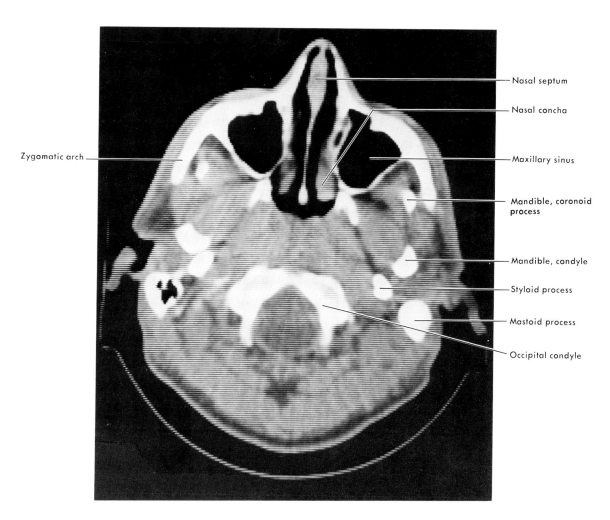

Nasal septum

Nasal concha

Zygomatic arch

Maxillary sinus

Mandible, coronoid process

Mandible, condyle

Styloid process

Mastoid process

Occipital condyle

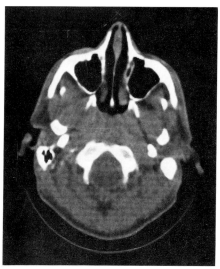

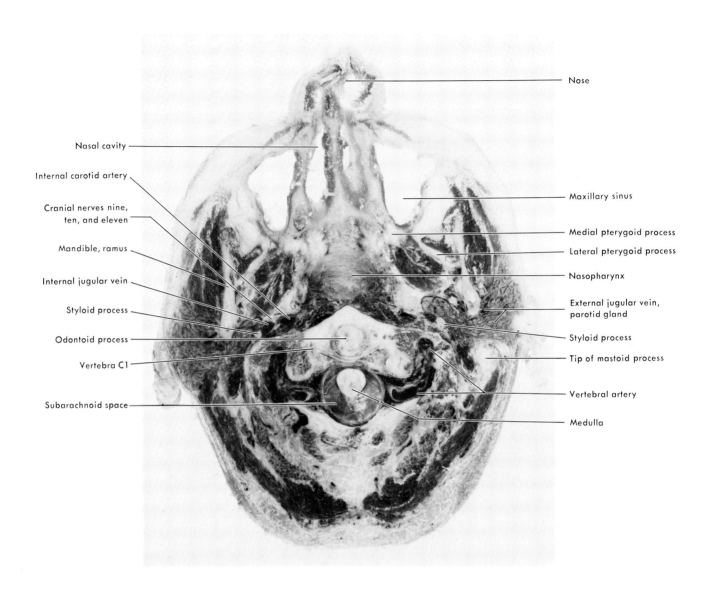

Nose

Nasal cavity

Internal carotid artery

Cranial nerves nine,
ten, and eleven

Mandible, ramus

Internal jugular vein

Styloid process

Odontoid process

Vertebra C1

Subarachnoid space

Maxillary sinus

Medial pterygoid process

Lateral pterygoid process

Nasopharynx

External jugular vein,
parotid gland

Styloid process

Tip of mastoid process

Vertebral artery

Medulla

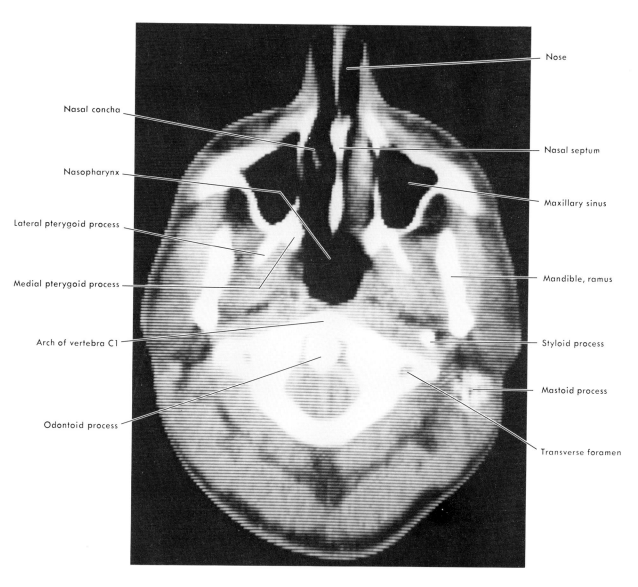

Nose

Nasal concha

Nasal septum

Nasopharynx

Maxillary sinus

Lateral pterygoid process

Medial pterygoid process

Mandible, ramus

Arch of vertebra C1

Styloid process

Mastoid process

Odontoid process

Transverse foramen

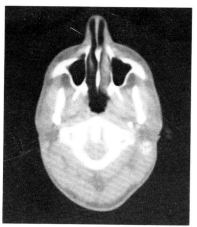

Computed tomography of the human body

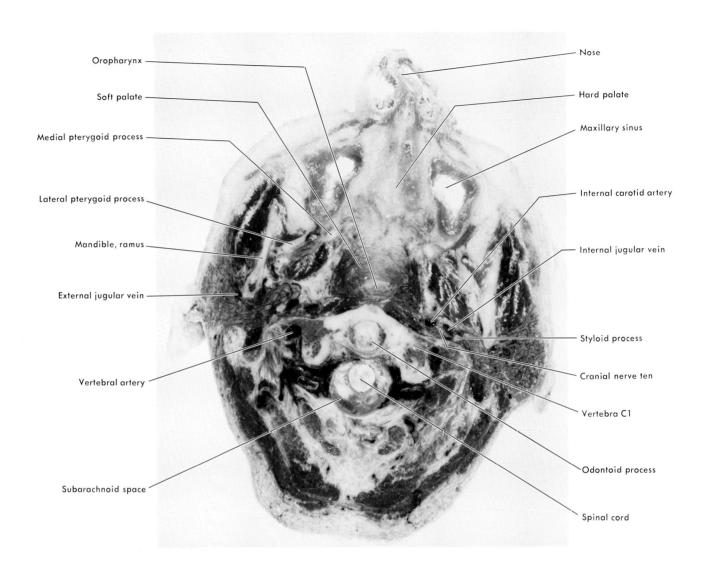

Oropharynx

Soft palate

Medial pterygoid process

Lateral pterygoid process

Mandible, ramus

External jugular vein

Vertebral artery

Subarachnoid space

Nose

Hard palate

Maxillary sinus

Internal carotid artery

Internal jugular vein

Styloid process

Cranial nerve ten

Vertebra C1

Odontoid process

Spinal cord

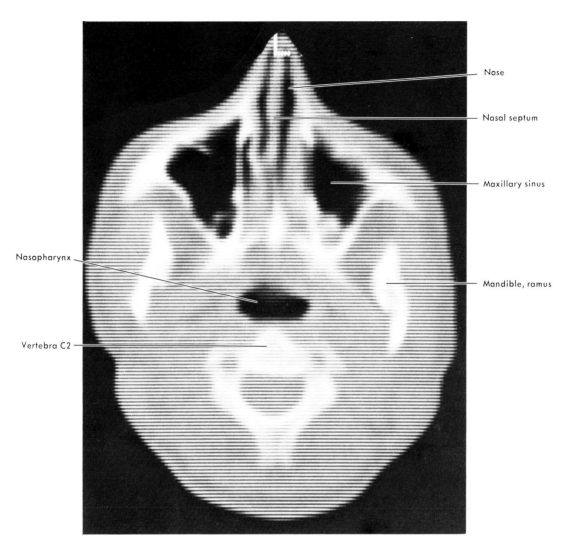

Nose

Nasal septum

Maxillary sinus

Nasopharynx

Mandible, ramus

Vertebra C2

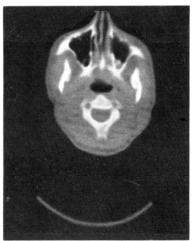

Computed tomography of the human body

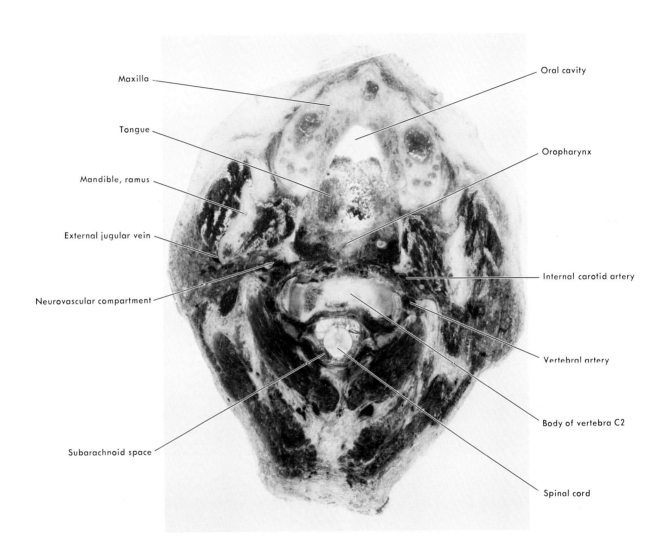

Maxilla

Tongue

Mandible, ramus

External jugular vein

Neurovascular compartment

Subarachnoid space

Oral cavity

Oropharynx

Internal carotid artery

Vertebral artery

Body of vertebra C2

Spinal cord

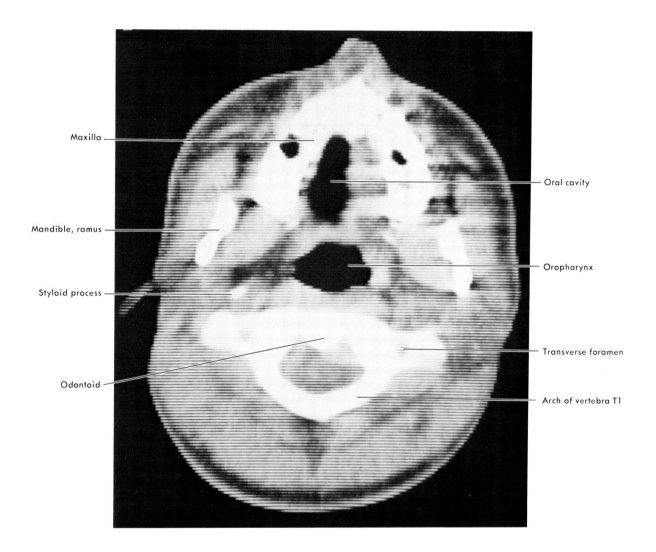

Maxilla

Mandible, ramus

Styloid process

Odontoid

Oral cavity

Oropharynx

Transverse foramen

Arch of vertebra T1

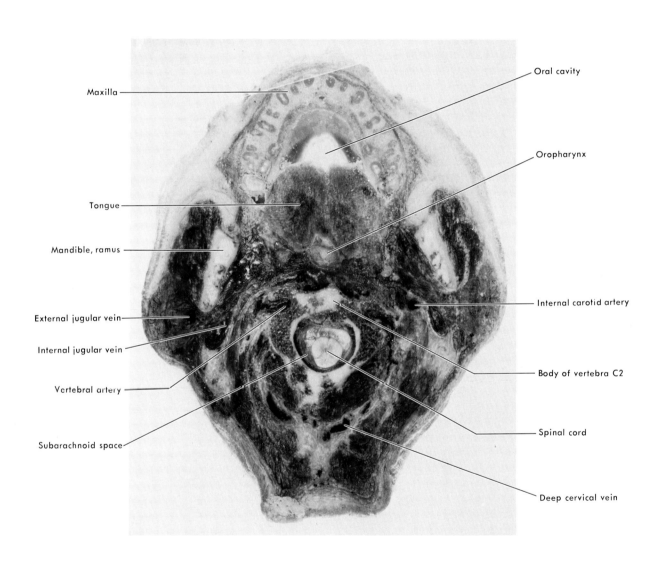

Maxilla

Tongue

Mandible, ramus

External jugular vein

Internal jugular vein

Vertebral artery

Subarachnoid space

Oral cavity

Oropharynx

Internal carotid artery

Body of vertebra C2

Spinal cord

Deep cervical vein

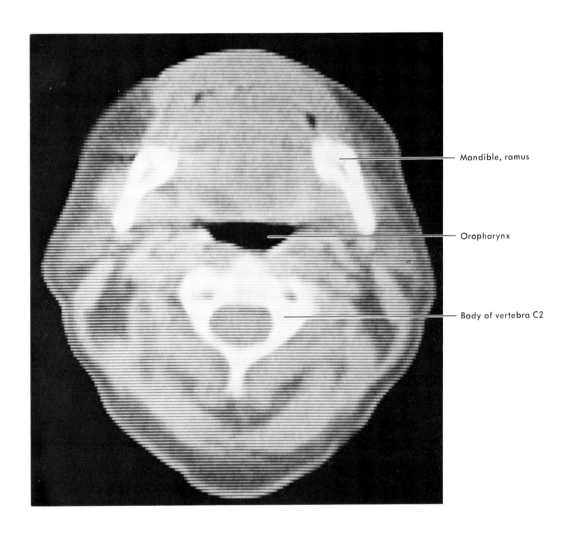

Mandible, ramus

Oropharynx

Body of vertebra C2

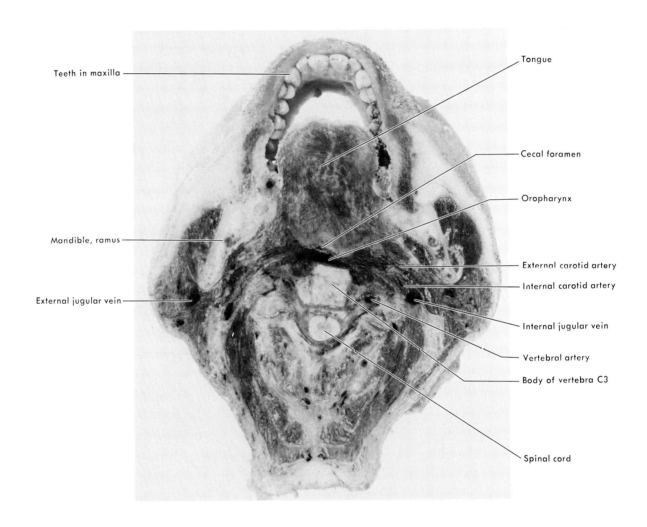

Teeth in maxilla

Tongue

Cecal foramen

Oropharynx

Mandible, ramus

External carotid artery

Internal carotid artery

External jugular vein

Internal jugular vein

Vertebral artery

Body of vertebra C3

Spinal cord

Mandible, ramus ——

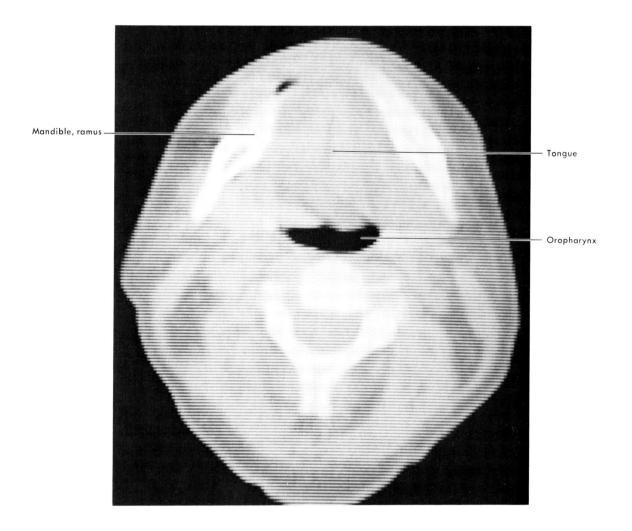

Tongue

Oropharynx

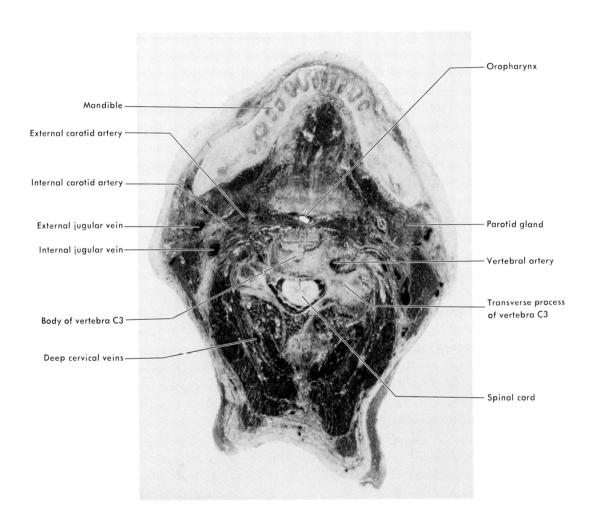

Mandible

External carotid artery

Internal carotid artery

External jugular vein

Internal jugular vein

Body of vertebra C3

Deep cervical veins

Oropharynx

Parotid gland

Vertebral artery

Transverse process of vertebra C3

Spinal cord

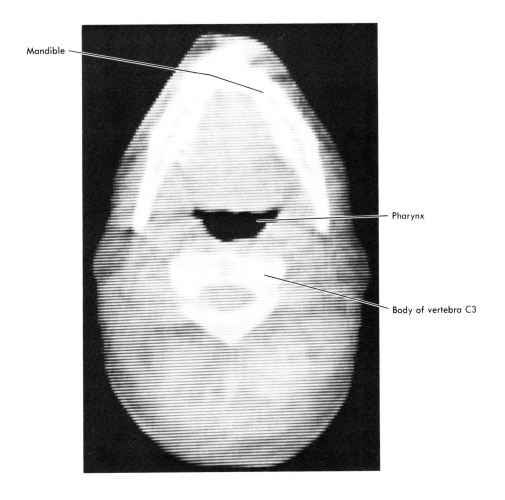

Mandible

Pharynx

Body of vertebra C3

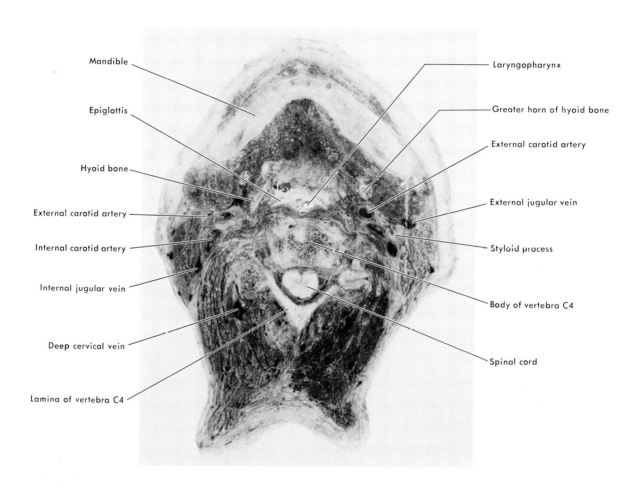

Mandible

Epiglottis

Hyoid bone

External carotid artery

Internal carotid artery

Internal jugular vein

Deep cervical vein

Lamina of vertebra C4

Laryngopharynx

Greater horn of hyoid bone

External carotid artery

External jugular vein

Styloid process

Body of vertebra C4

Spinal cord

Mandible

Hyoid bone

Pharynx

Transverse foramen

Lamina of vertebra C4

Spinal cord

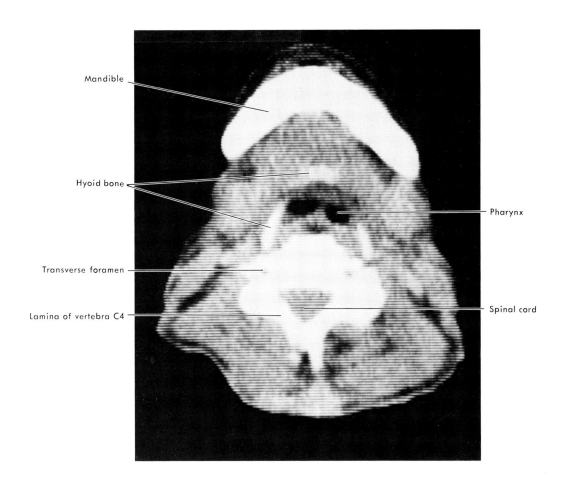

Internal jugular vein   Common carotid artery   Laryngeal vestibulum   Thyroid cartilage   Esophagus   Body of vertebra   Spinal cord   Clavicle   Humeral head

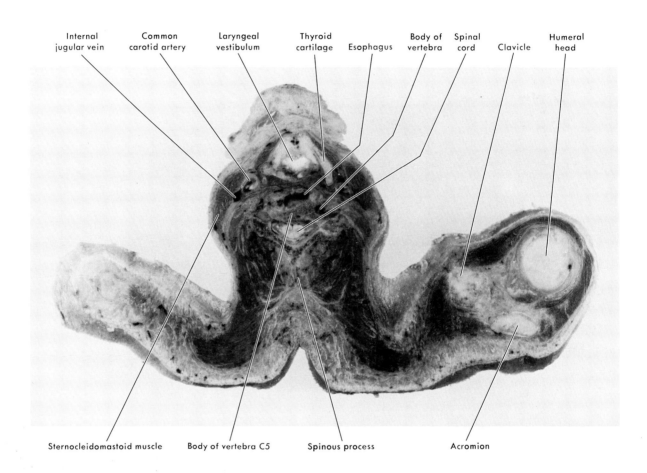

Sternocleidomastoid muscle   Body of vertebra C5   Spinous process   Acromion

Laryngeal cavity   Thyroid cartilage

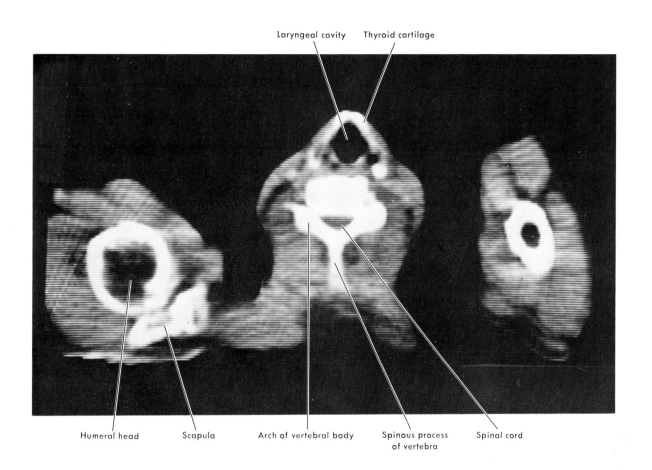

Humeral head   Scapula   Arch of vertebral body   Spinous process   Spinal cord
                                                      of vertebra

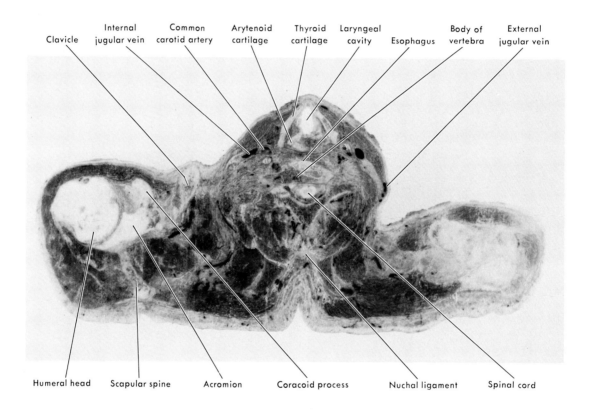

Clavicle   Internal jugular vein   Common carotid artery   Arytenoid cartilage   Thyroid cartilage   Laryngeal cavity   Esophagus   Body of vertebra   External jugular vein

Humeral head   Scapular spine   Acromion   Coracoid process   Nuchal ligament   Spinal cord

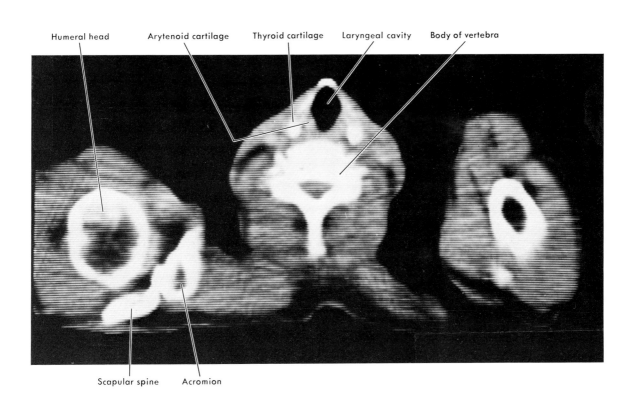

Humeral head   Arytenoid cartilage   Thyroid cartilage   Laryngeal cavity   Body of vertebra

Scapular spine   Acromion

Internal jugular vein | Body of vertebra C6 | Arytenoid cartilage | Rima glottidis | Thyroid cartilage | Common carotid artery | Transverse process of vertebra C6 | Clavicle | Coracoid process | Biceps tendon groove

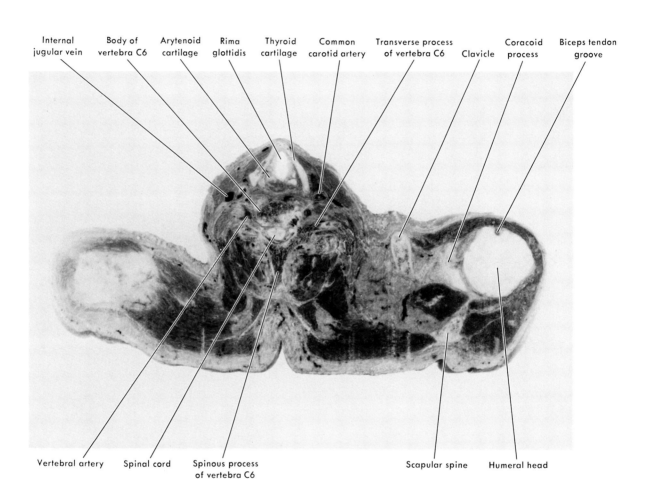

Vertebral artery | Spinal cord | Spinous process of vertebra C6 | Scapular spine | Humeral head

Body of vertebra C6   Arytenoid cartilage   Rima glottidis   Thyroid cartilage   Transverse process of vertebra C6

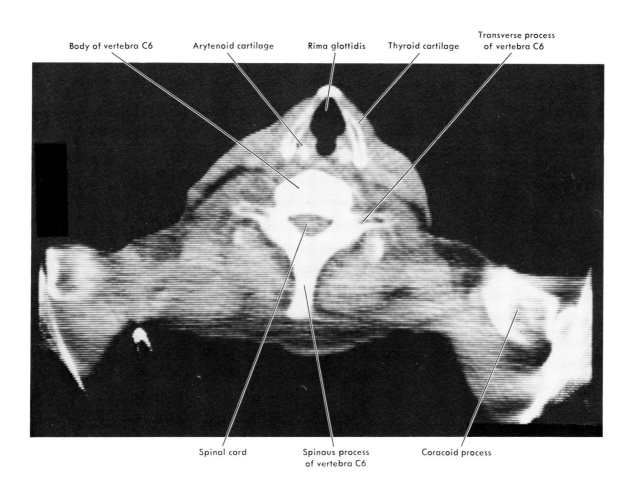

Spinal cord   Spinous process of vertebra C6   Coracoid process

Computed tomography of the human body

Clavicle Esophagus Tracheal ring Trachea Thyroid gland Common carotid artery Internal jugular vein Vertebral artery Coracoid process

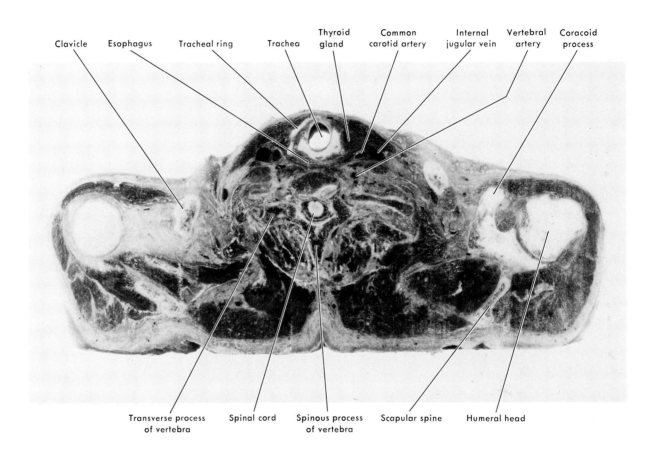

Transverse process of vertebra Spinal cord Spinous process of vertebra Scapular spine Humeral head

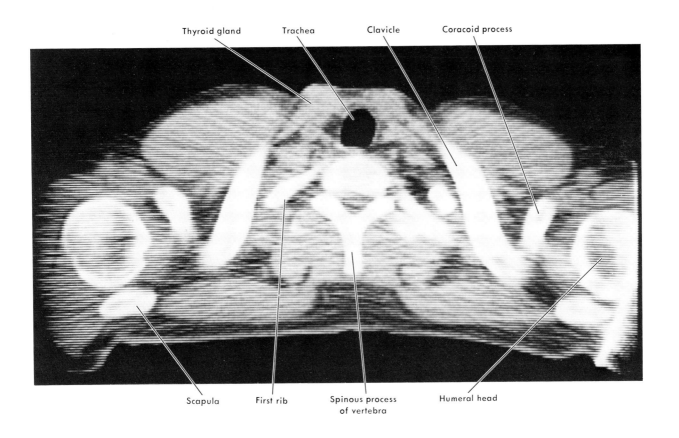

Thyroid gland   Trachea   Clavicle   Coracoid process

Scapula   First rib   Spinous process   Humeral head
                         of vertebra

Computed tomography of the human body

Humeral head Base of coracoid process Internal jugular vein Common carotid artery Thyroid gland Trachea Esophagus Body of vertebra T1 Clavicle Subclavian artery

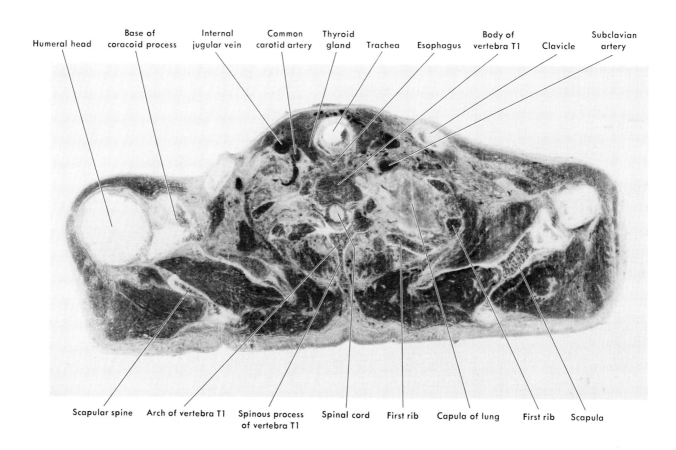

Scapular spine Arch of vertebra T1 Spinous process of vertebra T1 Spinal cord First rib Capula of lung First rib Scapula

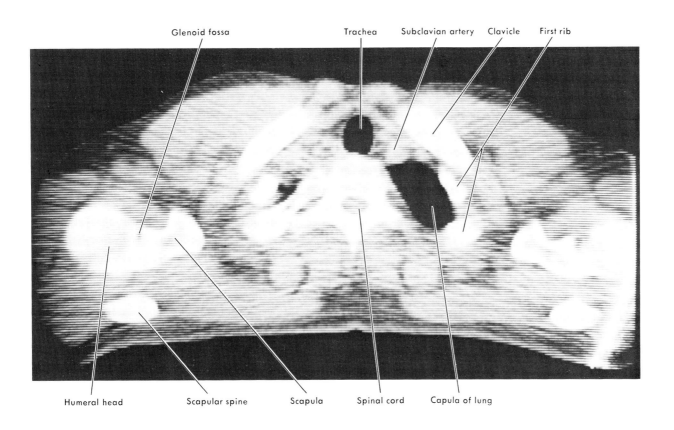

Glenoid fossa   Trachea   Subclavian artery   Clavicle   First rib

Humeral head   Scapular spine   Scapula   Spinal cord   Capula of lung

Chapter 3

CHEST

RALPH ALFIDI
JOHN HAAGA

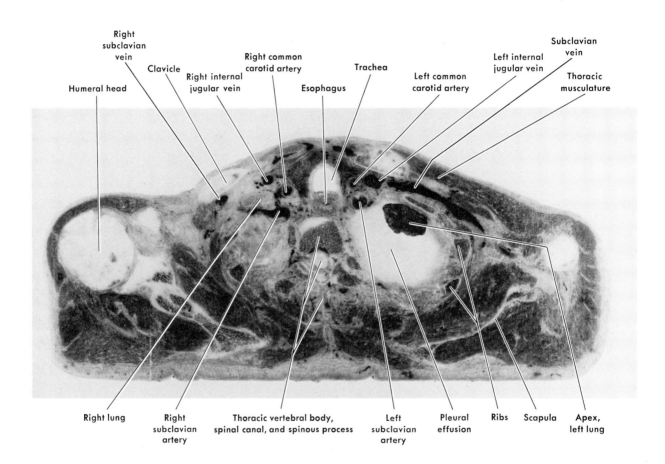

Right subclavian vein

Clavicle

Humeral head

Right internal jugular vein

Right common carotid artery

Esophagus

Trachea

Left common carotid artery

Left internal jugular vein

Subclavian vein

Thoracic musculature

Right lung

Right subclavian artery

Thoracic vertebral body, spinal canal, and spinous process

Left subclavian artery

Pleural effusion

Ribs

Scapula

Apex, left lung

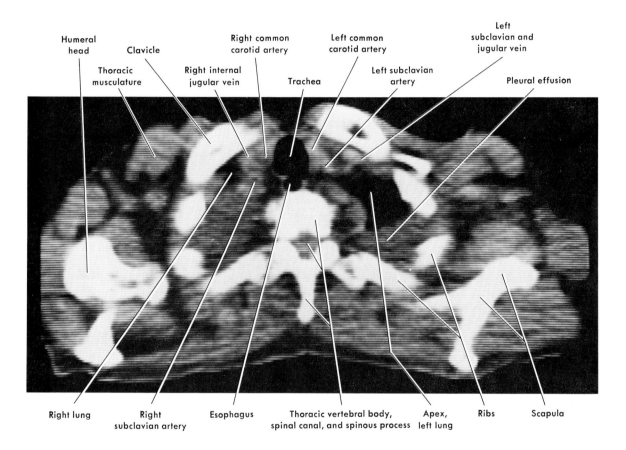

Humeral
head

Clavicle

Thoracic
musculature

Right internal
jugular vein

Right common
carotid artery

Trachea

Left common
carotid artery

Left subclavian
artery

Left
subclavian and
jugular vein

Pleural effusion

Right lung

Right
subclavian artery

Esophagus

Thoracic vertebral body,
spinal canal, and spinous process

Apex,
left lung

Ribs

Scapula

Computed tomography of the human body

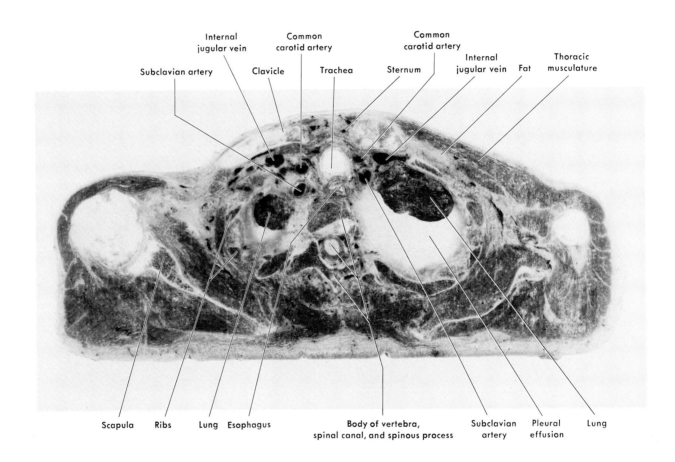

Internal jugular vein

Common carotid artery

Common carotid artery

Subclavian artery

Clavicle

Trachea

Sternum

Internal jugular vein

Fat

Thoracic musculature

Scapula   Ribs   Lung   Esophagus

Body of vertebra, spinal canal, and spinous process

Subclavian artery

Pleural effusion

Lung

Ascending aorta   Sternum   Mediastinal fat   Left pulmonary artery

Anterior
mediastinal fat

Superior vena cava   Mediastinal lymph node   Esophagus   Thoracic musculature

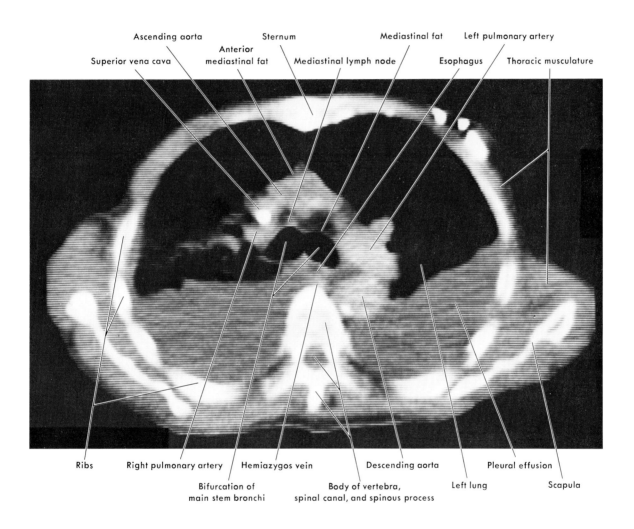

Ribs   Right pulmonary artery   Hemiazygos vein   Descending aorta   Pleural effusion   Scapula

Bifurcation of
main stem bronchi

Body of vertebra,
spinal canal, and spinous process   Left lung

Computed tomography of the human body

Right lung   Superior vena cava   Anterior mediastinal fat   Esophagus   Skin

Right pulmonary artery   Ascending aorta   Sternum   Left pulmonary artery   Thoracic musculature

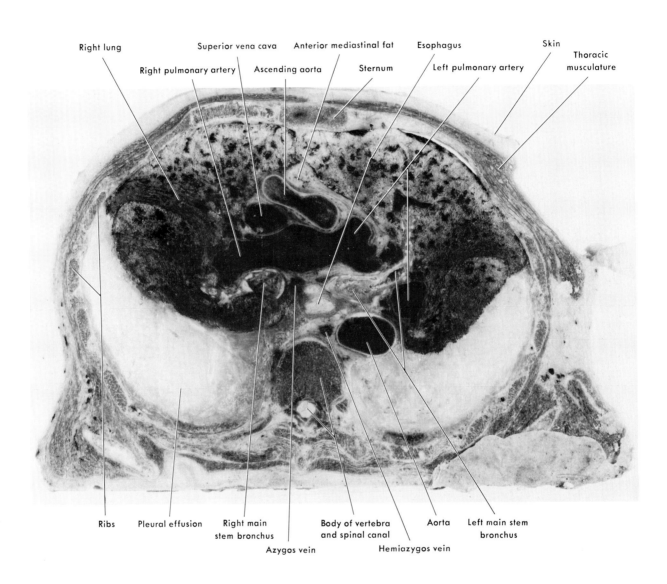

Ribs   Pleural effusion   Right main stem bronchus   Body of vertebra and spinal canal   Aorta   Left main stem bronchus

Azygos vein   Hemiazygos vein

Ribs

Right lung

Superior vena cava

Anterior mediastinal fat

Esophagus

Skin

Right pulmonary artery

Ascending aorta

Sternum

Left pulmonary artery

Thoracic musculature

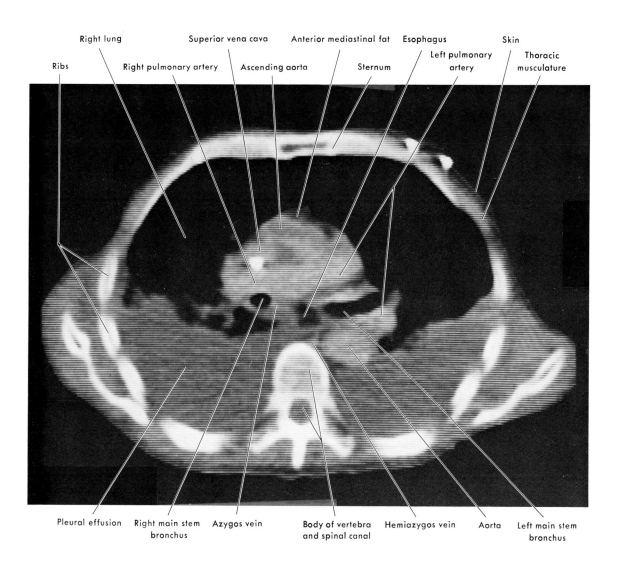

Pleural effusion

Right main stem bronchus

Azygos vein

Body of vertebra and spinal canal

Hemiazygos vein

Aorta

Left main stem bronchus

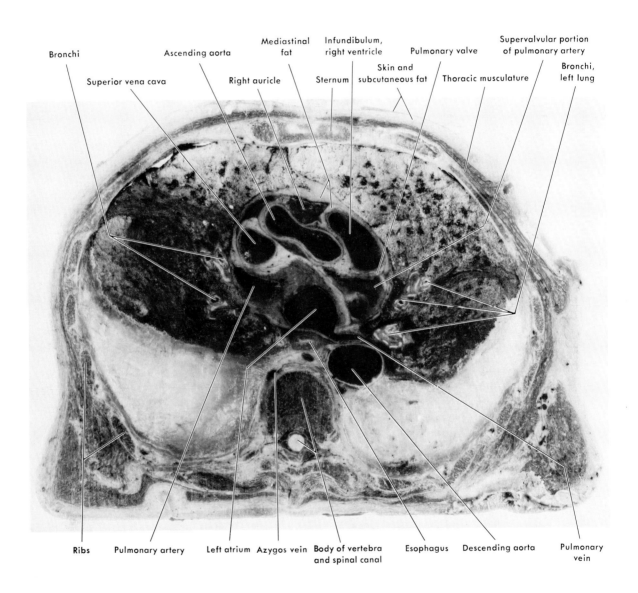

Bronchi   Ascending aorta   Mediastinal fat   Infundibulum, right ventricle   Pulmonary valve   Supervalvular portion of pulmonary artery

Superior vena cava   Right auricle   Sternum   Skin and subcutaneous fat   Thoracic musculature   Bronchi, left lung

Ribs   Pulmonary artery   Left atrium   Azygos vein   Body of vertebra and spinal canal   Esophagus   Descending aorta   Pulmonary vein

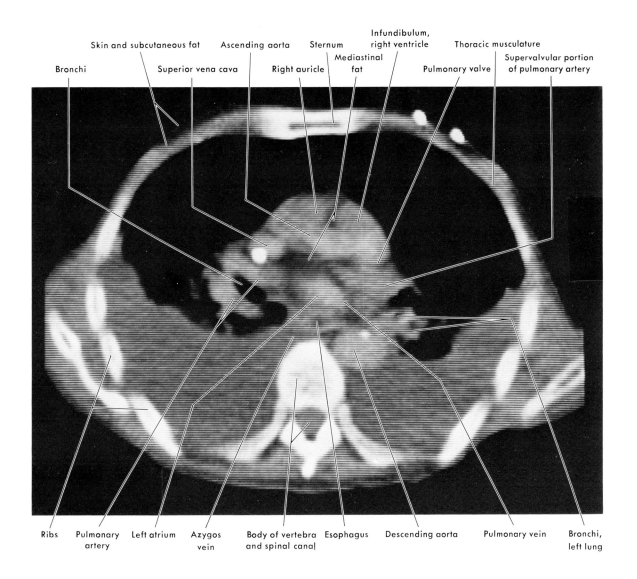

Bronchi

Skin and subcutaneous fat

Superior vena cava

Ascending aorta

Right auricle

Sternum

Mediastinal fat

Infundibulum, right ventricle

Pulmonary valve

Thoracic musculature

Supervalvular portion of pulmonary artery

Ribs

Pulmonary artery

Left atrium

Azygos vein

Body of vertebra and spinal canal

Esophagus

Descending aorta

Pulmonary vein

Bronchi, left lung

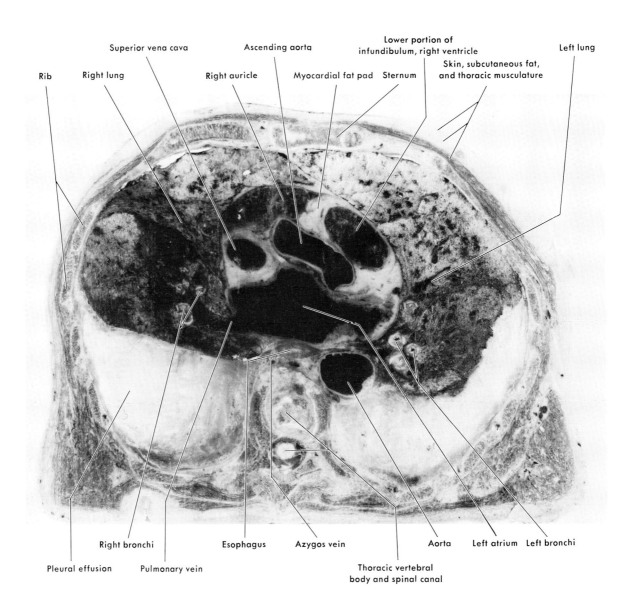

Rib Right lung Superior vena cava Right auricle Ascending aorta Myocardial fat pad Sternum Lower portion of infundibulum, right ventricle Skin, subcutaneous fat, and thoracic musculature Left lung

Pleural effusion Right bronchi Pulmonary vein Esophagus Azygos vein Thoracic vertebral body and spinal canal Aorta Left atrium Left bronchi

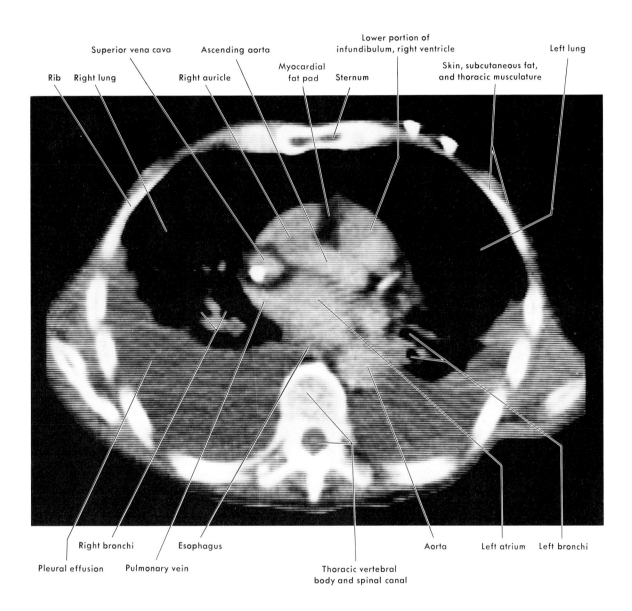

Rib Right lung

Superior vena cava

Ascending aorta

Right auricle

Myocardial
fat pad

Lower portion of
infundibulum, right ventricle

Sternum

Left lung

Skin, subcutaneous fat,
and thoracic musculature

Right bronchi

Esophagus

Pleural effusion

Pulmonary vein

Thoracic vertebral
body and spinal canal

Aorta

Left atrium

Left bronchi

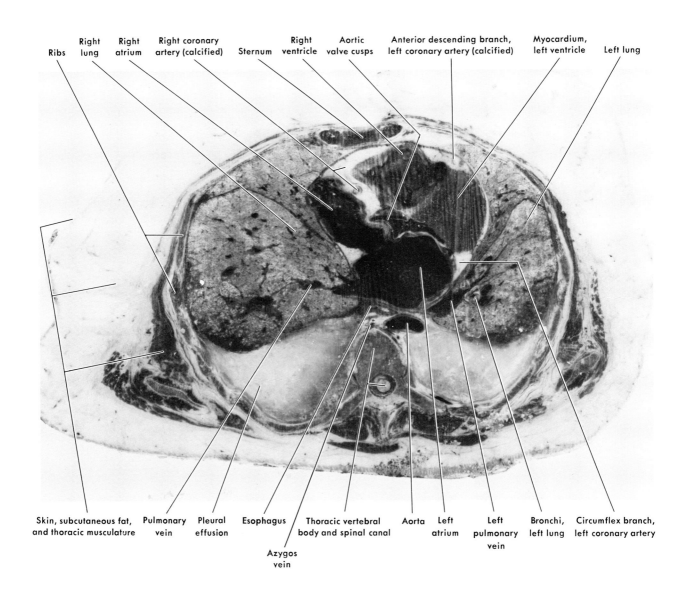

Ribs · Right lung · Right atrium · Right coronary artery (calcified) · Sternum · Right ventricle · Aortic valve cusps · Anterior descending branch, left coronary artery (calcified) · Myocardium, left ventricle · Left lung

Skin, subcutaneous fat, and thoracic musculature · Pulmonary vein · Pleural effusion · Esophagus · Thoracic vertebral body and spinal canal · Aorta · Left atrium · Left pulmonary vein · Bronchi, left lung · Circumflex branch, left coronary artery

Azygos vein

Right   Right   Right coronary   Right   Aortic   Anterior descending branch,   Myocardium,   Left
Ribs   lung   atrium   artery (calcified)   Sternum   ventricle   valve cusps   left coronary artery (calcified)   left ventricle   lung

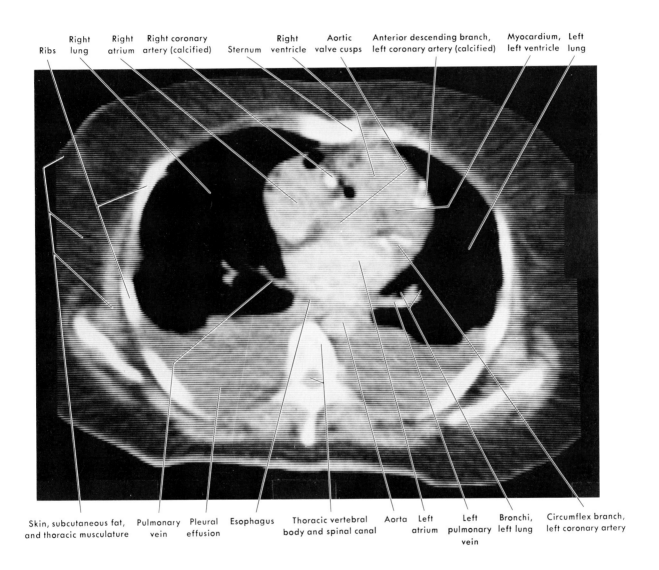

Skin, subcutaneous fat,   Pulmonary   Pleural   Esophagus   Thoracic vertebral   Aorta   Left   Left   Bronchi,   Circumflex branch,
and thoracic musculature   vein   effusion   body and spinal canal   atrium   pulmonary   left lung   left coronary artery
    vein

Computed tomography of the human body

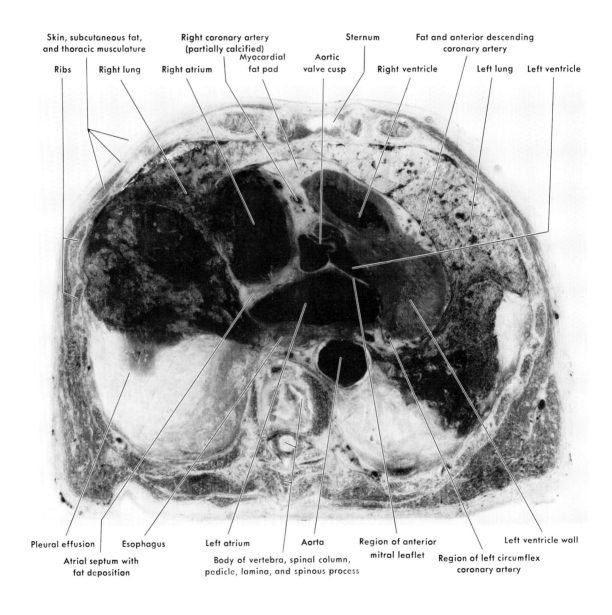

Skin, subcutaneous fat, and thoracic musculature

Ribs   Right lung   Right atrium

Right coronary artery (partially calcified)

Myocardial fat pad

Aortic valve cusp

Sternum

Right ventricle

Fat and anterior descending coronary artery

Left lung   Left ventricle

Pleural effusion   Esophagus   Left atrium   Aorta   Region of anterior mitral leaflet   Left ventricle wall

Atrial septum with fat deposition

Body of vertebra, spinal column, pedicle, lamina, and spinous process

Region of left circumflex coronary artery

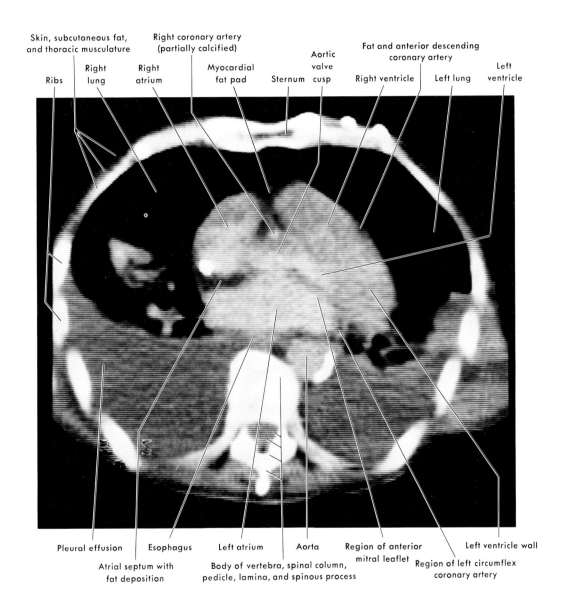

Skin, subcutaneous fat, and thoracic musculature

Ribs

Right lung

Right atrium

Right coronary artery (partially calcified)

Myocardial fat pad

Sternum

Aortic valve cusp

Fat and anterior descending coronary artery

Right ventricle

Left lung

Left ventricle

Pleural effusion

Atrial septum with fat deposition

Esophagus

Left atrium

Body of vertebra, spinal column, pedicle, lamina, and spinous process

Aorta

Region of anterior mitral leaflet

Region of left circumflex coronary artery

Left ventricle wall

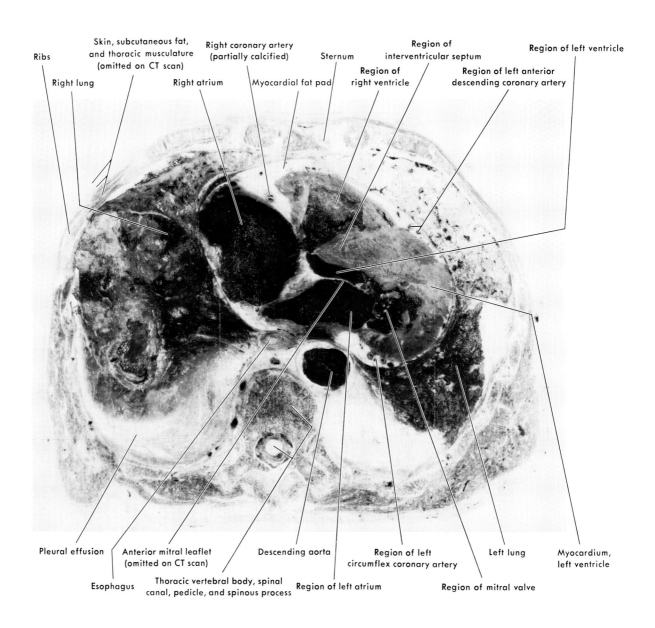

Ribs

Skin, subcutaneous fat, and thoracic musculature (omitted on CT scan)

Right coronary artery (partially calcified)

Sternum

Region of interventricular septum

Region of left ventricle

Right lung

Right atrium

Myocardial fat pad

Region of right ventricle

Region of left anterior descending coronary artery

Pleural effusion

Anterior mitral leaflet (omitted on CT scan)

Descending aorta

Region of left circumflex coronary artery

Left lung

Myocardium, left ventricle

Esophagus

Thoracic vertebral body, spinal canal, pedicle, and spinous process

Region of left atrium

Region of mitral valve

Right coronary artery
(partially calcified)

Sternum

Region of
interventricular septum

Region of left ventricle

Region of left anterior
descending coronary artery

Ribs   Right lung   Right atrium   Myocardial fat pad

Region of
right ventricle

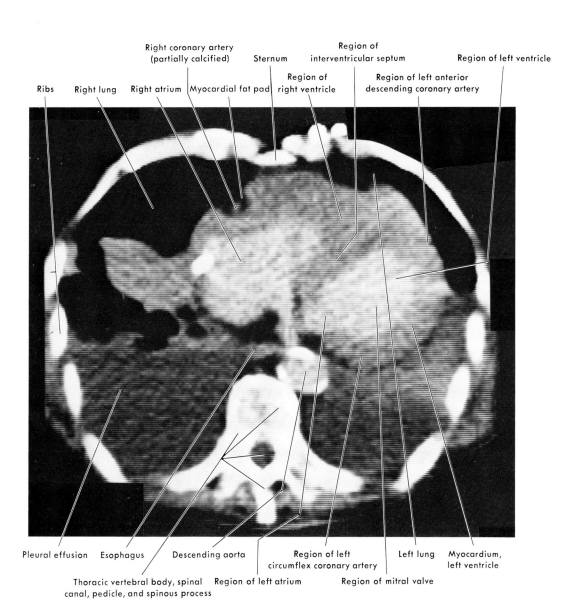

Pleural effusion   Esophagus   Descending aorta

Region of left
circumflex coronary artery

Left lung

Myocardium,
left ventricle

Thoracic vertebral body, spinal
canal, pedicle, and spinous process

Region of left atrium

Region of mitral valve

Computed tomography of the human body

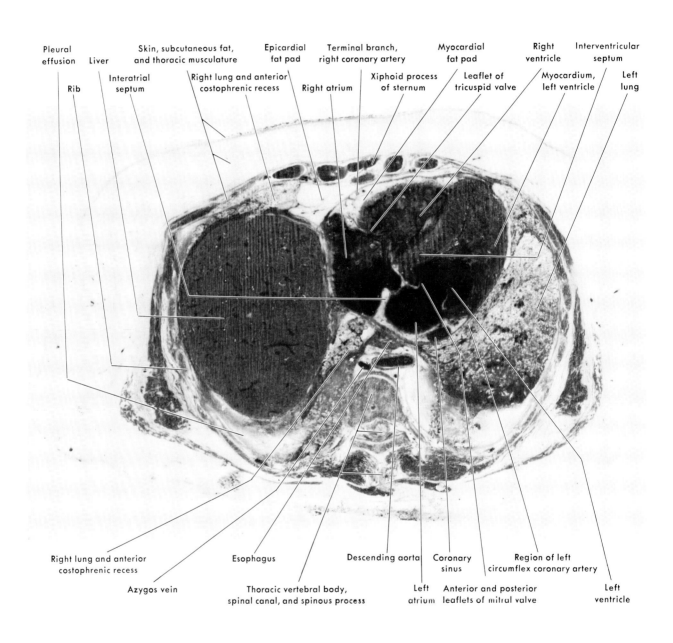

Pleural effusion | Liver | Skin, subcutaneous fat, and thoracic musculature | Epicardial fat pad | Terminal branch, right coronary artery | Myocardial fat pad | Right ventricle | Interventricular septum

Rib | Interatrial septum | Right lung and anterior costophrenic recess | Right atrium | Xiphoid process of sternum | Leaflet of tricuspid valve | Myocardium, left ventricle | Left lung

Right lung and anterior costophrenic recess | Esophagus | Descending aorta | Coronary sinus | Region of left circumflex coronary artery | Left ventricle

Azygos vein | Thoracic vertebral body, spinal canal, and spinous process | Left atrium | Anterior and posterior leaflets of mitral valve

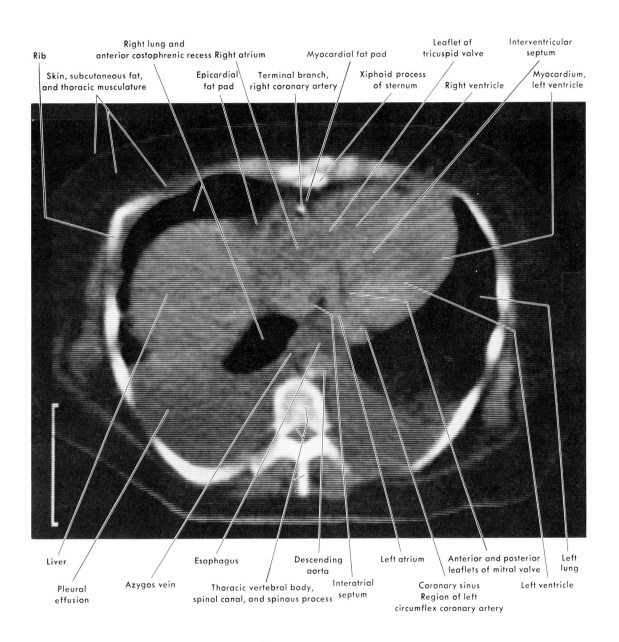

Rib

Right lung and
anterior costophrenic recess Right atrium

Myocardial fat pad

Leaflet of
tricuspid valve

Interventricular
septum

Skin, subcutaneous fat,
and thoracic musculature

Epicardial
fat pad

Terminal branch,
right coronary artery

Xiphoid process
of sternum

Right ventricle

Myocardium,
left ventricle

Liver

Pleural
effusion

Azygos vein

Esophagus

Thoracic vertebral body,
spinal canal, and spinous process

Descending
aorta

Interatrial
septum

Left atrium

Coronary sinus
Region of left
circumflex coronary artery

Anterior and posterior
leaflets of mitral valve

Left
lung

Left ventricle

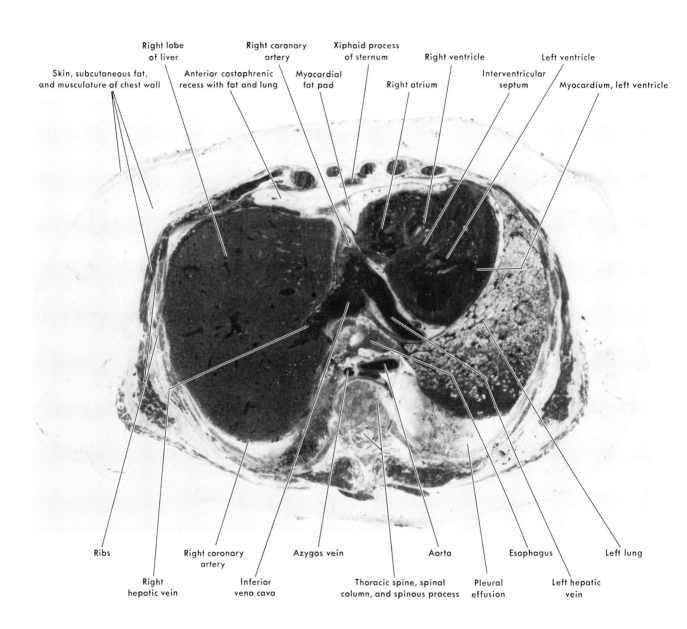

Skin, subcutaneous fat, and musculature of chest wall — Right lobe of liver — Anterior costophrenic recess with fat and lung — Right coronary artery — Myocardial fat pad — Xiphoid process of sternum — Right atrium — Right ventricle — Interventricular septum — Left ventricle — Myocardium, left ventricle

Ribs — Right hepatic vein — Right coronary artery — Inferior vena cava — Azygos vein — Thoracic spine, spinal column, and spinous process — Aorta — Pleural effusion — Esophagus — Left hepatic vein — Left lung

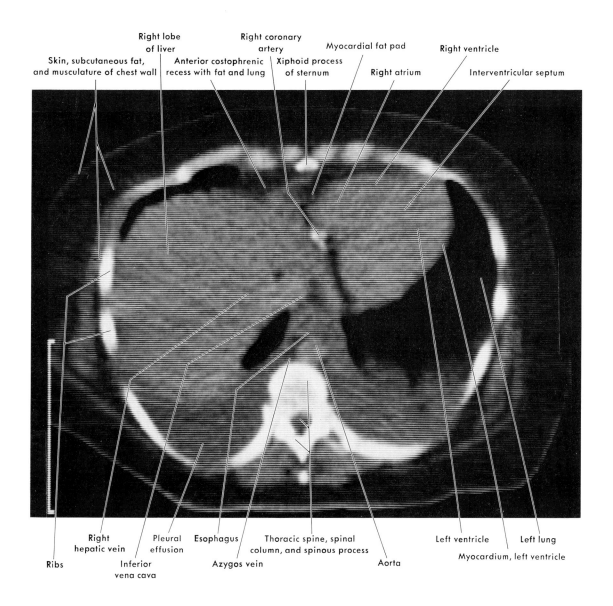

Skin, subcutaneous fat, and musculature of chest wall

Right lobe of liver

Anterior costophrenic recess with fat and lung

Right coronary artery

Xiphoid process of sternum

Myocardial fat pad

Right atrium

Right ventricle

Interventricular septum

Ribs

Right hepatic vein

Inferior vena cava

Pleural effusion

Esophagus

Azygos vein

Thoracic spine, spinal column, and spinous process

Aorta

Left ventricle

Myocardium, left ventricle

Left lung

Chapter 4

ABDOMEN

RALPH ALFIDI
JOHN HAAGA

Computed tomography of the human body

Ribs Right lobe of liver Diaphragm Caudate lobe of liver Left lobe of liver Vena cava Aorta Stomach Spleen

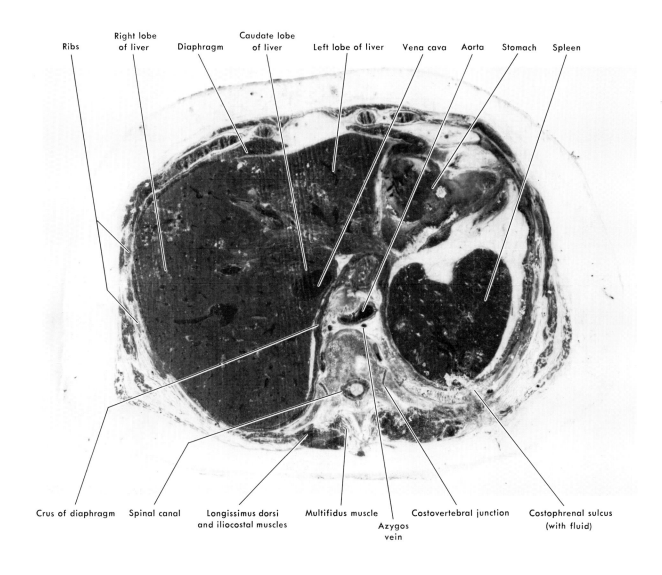

Crus of diaphragm Spinal canal Longissimus dorsi and iliocostal muscles Multifidus muscle Azygos vein Costovertebral junction Costophrenal sulcus (with fluid)

Vena cava   Right lobe of liver   Caudate lobe of liver   Left lobe of liver   Diaphragm   Stomach   Spleen   Ribs

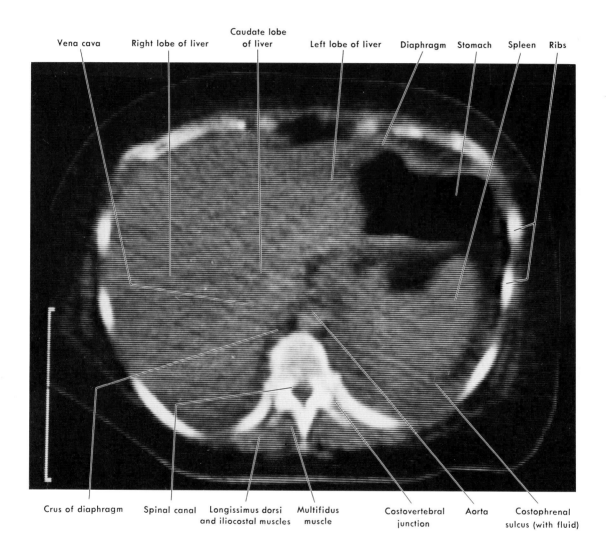

Crus of diaphragm   Spinal canal   Longissimus dorsi and iliocostal muscles   Multifidus muscle   Costovertebral junction   Aorta   Costophrenal sulcus (with fluid)

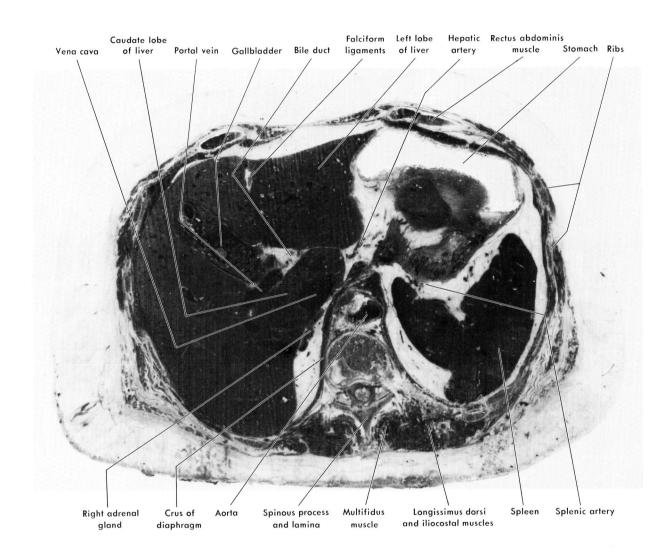

Vena cava · Caudate lobe of liver · Portal vein · Gallbladder · Bile duct · Falciform ligaments · Left lobe of liver · Hepatic artery · Rectus abdominis muscle · Stomach · Ribs

Right adrenal gland · Crus of diaphragm · Aorta · Spinous process and lamina · Multifidus muscle · Longissimus dorsi and iliocostal muscles · Spleen · Splenic artery

Caudate lobe of liver

Vena cava   Portal vein   Gallbladder   Bile duct   Falciform ligaments   Left lobe of liver   Hepatic artery   Rectus abdominis muscle   Stomach   Ribs

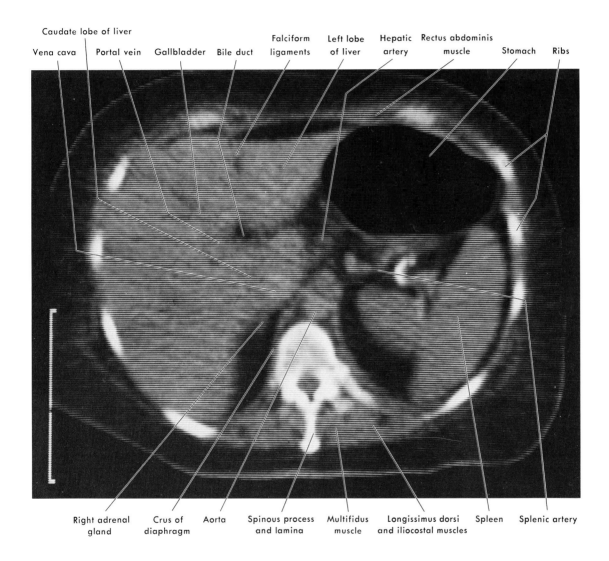

Right adrenal gland   Crus of diaphragm   Aorta   Spinous process and lamina   Multifidus muscle   Longissimus dorsi and iliocostal muscles   Spleen   Splenic artery

137

Computed tomography of the human body

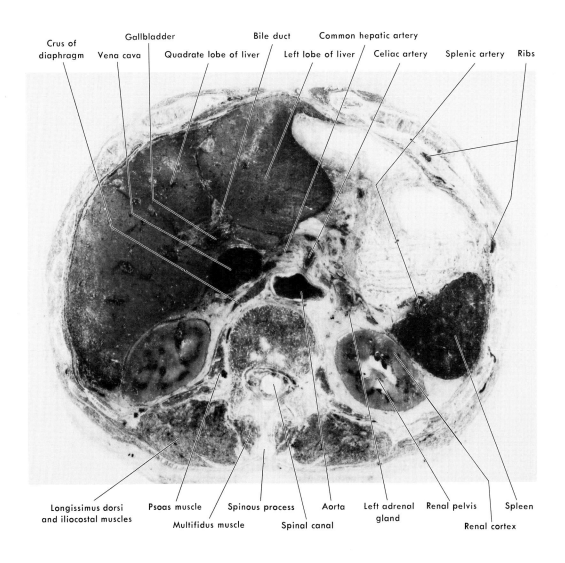

Crus of diaphragm   Vena cava   Gallbladder   Quadrate lobe of liver   Bile duct   Left lobe of liver   Common hepatic artery   Celiac artery   Splenic artery   Ribs

Longissimus dorsi and iliocostal muscles   Psoas muscle   Multifidus muscle   Spinous process   Spinal canal   Aorta   Left adrenal gland   Renal pelvis   Renal cortex   Spleen

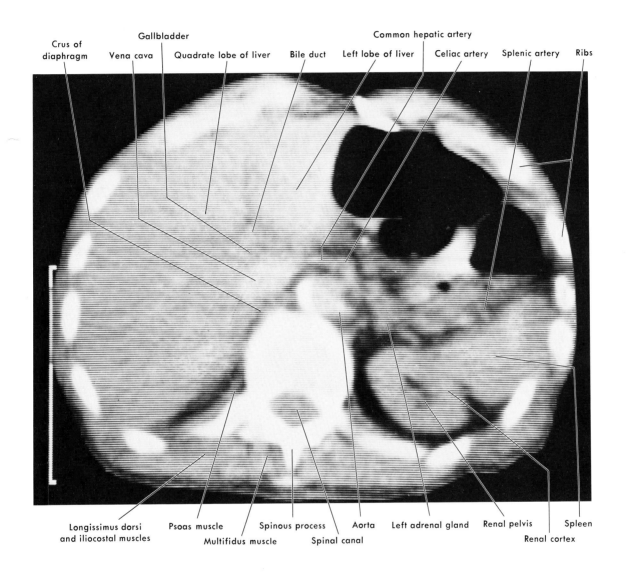

Crus of diaphragm

Gallbladder

Vena cava

Quadrate lobe of liver

Bile duct

Left lobe of liver

Common hepatic artery

Celiac artery

Splenic artery

Ribs

Longissimus dorsi and iliocostal muscles

Psoas muscle

Multifidus muscle

Spinous process

Spinal canal

Aorta

Left adrenal gland

Renal pelvis

Renal cortex

Spleen

Computed tomography of the human body

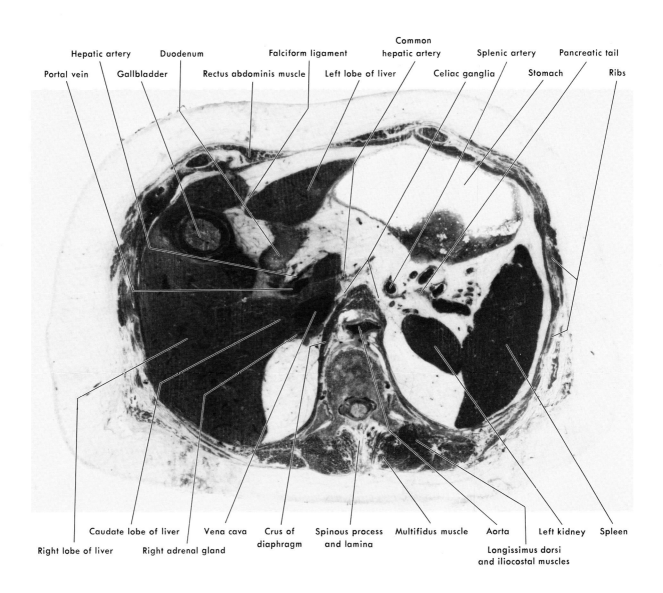

Hepatic artery

Portal vein

Duodenum

Gallbladder

Falciform ligament

Rectus abdominis muscle

Common
hepatic artery

Left lobe of liver

Celiac ganglia

Splenic artery

Stomach

Pancreatic tail

Ribs

Caudate lobe of liver

Right lobe of liver

Vena cava

Right adrenal gland

Crus of
diaphragm

Spinous process
and lamina

Multifidus muscle

Aorta

Longissimus dorsi
and iliocostal muscles

Left kidney

Spleen

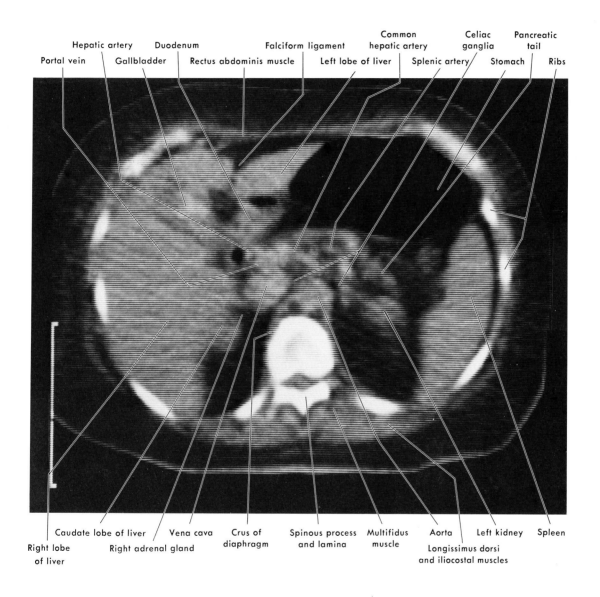

Portal vein

Hepatic artery

Gallbladder

Duodenum

Rectus abdominis muscle

Falciform ligament

Left lobe of liver

Common
hepatic artery

Splenic artery

Celiac
ganglia

Stomach

Pancreatic
tail

Ribs

Right lobe
of liver

Caudate lobe of liver

Right adrenal gland

Vena cava

Crus of
diaphragm

Spinous process
and lamina

Multifidus
muscle

Aorta

Longissimus dorsi
and iliocostal muscles

Left kidney

Spleen

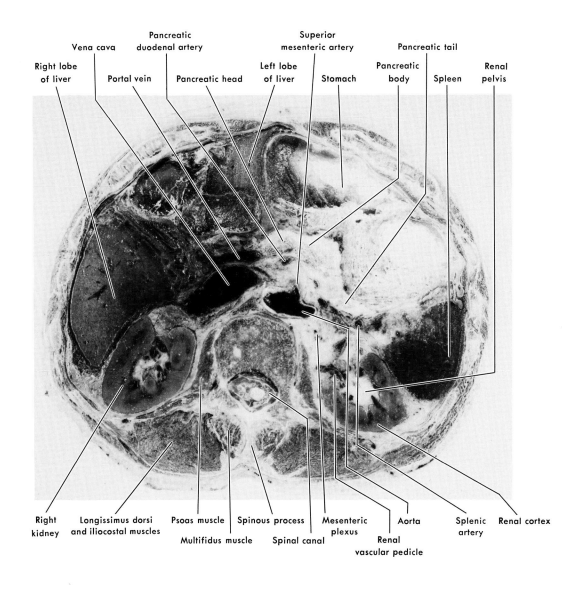

Right lobe of liver · Vena cava · Portal vein · Pancreatic duodenal artery · Pancreatic head · Left lobe of liver · Superior mesenteric artery · Stomach · Pancreatic body · Pancreatic tail · Spleen · Renal pelvis

Right kidney · Longissimus dorsi and iliocostal muscles · Psoas muscle · Multifidus muscle · Spinous process · Spinal canal · Mesenteric plexus · Renal vascular pedicle · Aorta · Splenic artery · Renal cortex

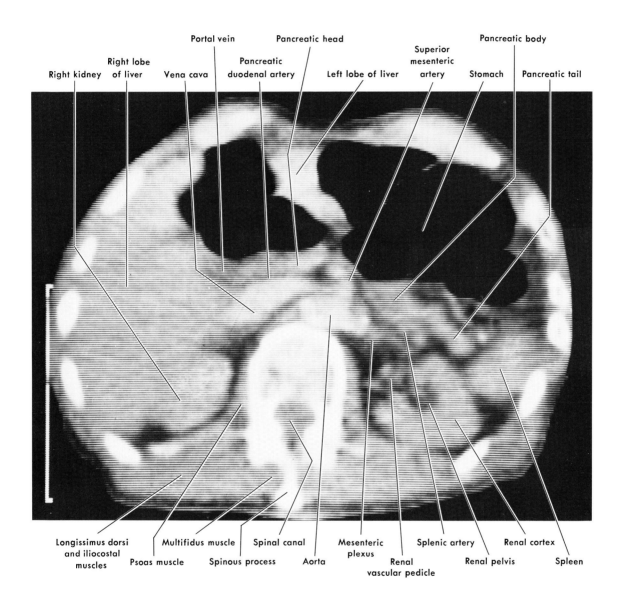

Portal vein   Pancreatic head   Pancreatic body

Right lobe   Pancreatic   Superior   mesenteric

Right kidney   of liver   Vena cava   duodenal artery   Left lobe of liver   artery   Stomach   Pancreatic tail

Longissimus dorsi   Multifidus muscle   Spinal canal   Mesenteric   Splenic artery   Renal cortex

and iliocostal   plexus

muscles   Psoas muscle   Spinous process   Aorta   Renal   Renal pelvis   Spleen

vascular pedicle

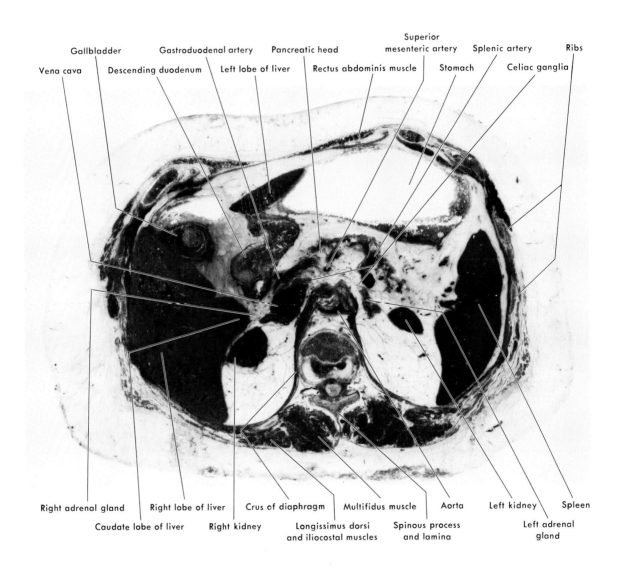

Gallbladder Gastroduodenal artery Pancreatic head Superior mesenteric artery Splenic artery Ribs

Vena cava Descending duodenum Left lobe of liver Rectus abdominis muscle Stomach Celiac ganglia

Right adrenal gland Right lobe of liver Crus of diaphragm Multifidus muscle Aorta Left kidney Spleen

Caudate lobe of liver Right kidney Longissimus dorsi and iliocostal muscles Spinous process and lamina Left adrenal gland

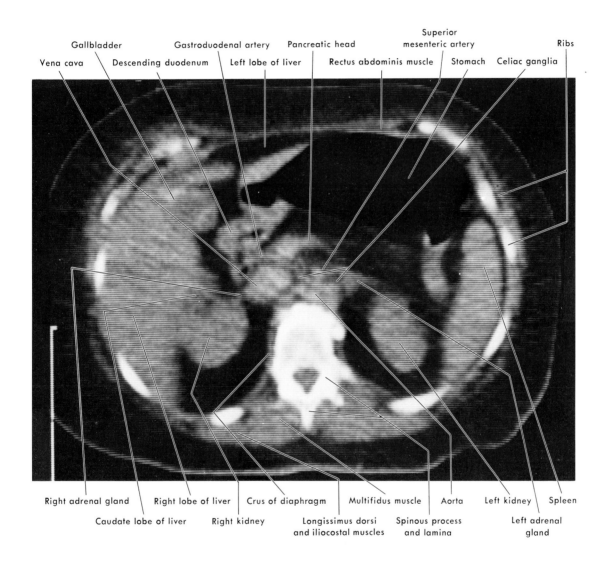

Gallbladder   Gastroduodenal artery   Pancreatic head   Superior mesenteric artery   Ribs

Vena cava   Descending duodenum   Left lobe of liver   Rectus abdominis muscle   Stomach   Celiac ganglia

Right adrenal gland   Right lobe of liver   Crus of diaphragm   Multifidus muscle   Aorta   Left kidney   Spleen

Caudate lobe of liver   Right kidney   Longissimus dorsi and iliocostal muscles   Spinous process and lamina   Left adrenal gland

Computed tomography of the human body

Right lobe of liver   Pancreatic head   Hepatic flexure of colon   Inferior portion of duodenum   Stomach   Superior mesenteric artery   Superior mesenteric plexus   Ribs   Spleen

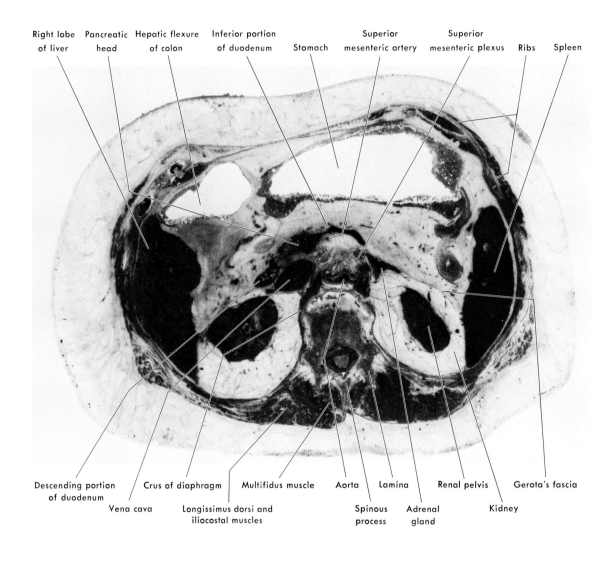

Descending portion of duodenum   Vena cava   Crus of diaphragm   Longissimus dorsi and iliocostal muscles   Multifidus muscle   Aorta   Spinous process   Lamina   Adrenal gland   Renal pelvis   Kidney   Gerota's fascia

146

Right lobe of liver   Pancreatic head   Hepatic flexure of colon   Inferior portion of duodenum   Stomach   Superior mesenteric artery   Superior mesenteric plexus   Ribs   Spleen

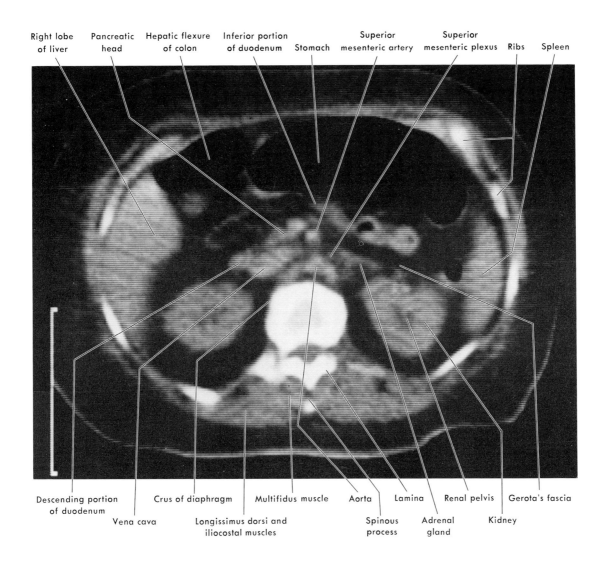

Descending portion of duodenum   Vena cava   Crus of diaphragm   Longissimus dorsi and iliocostal muscles   Multifidus muscle   Aorta   Spinous process   Lamina   Adrenal gland   Renal pelvis   Kidney   Gerota's fascia

Computed tomography of the human body

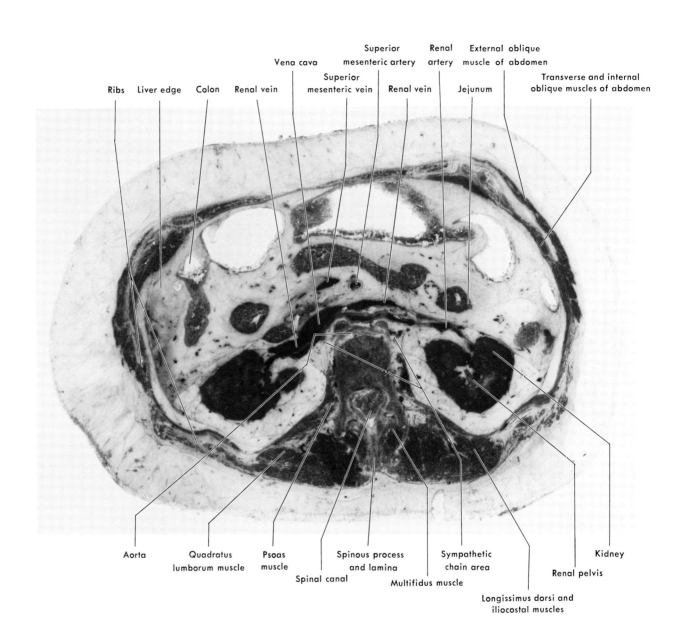

Ribs Liver edge Colon Renal vein Vena cava Superior mesenteric vein Superior mesenteric artery Renal vein Renal artery Jejunum External oblique muscle of abdomen Transverse and internal oblique muscles of abdomen

Aorta Quadratus lumborum muscle Psoas muscle Spinal canal Spinous process and lamina Multifidus muscle Sympathetic chain area Longissimus dorsi and iliocostal muscles Renal pelvis Kidney

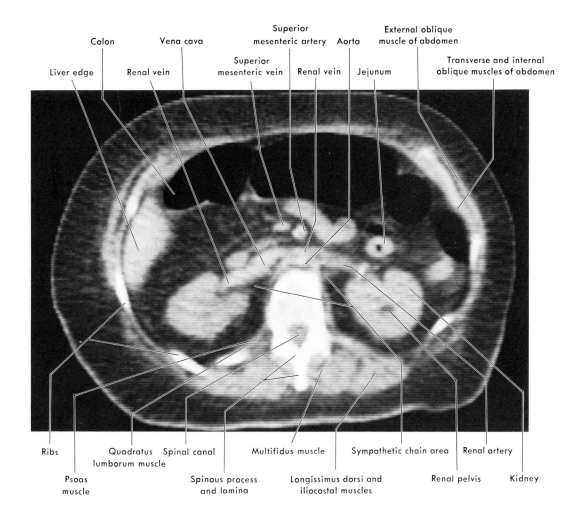

Colon Vena cava Superior mesenteric artery Aorta External oblique muscle of abdomen

Liver edge Renal vein Superior mesenteric vein Renal vein Jejunum Transverse and internal oblique muscles of abdomen

Ribs Quadratus lumborum muscle Spinal canal Multifidus muscle Sympathetic chain area Renal artery

Psoas muscle Spinous process and lamina Longissimus dorsi and iliocostal muscles Renal pelvis Kidney

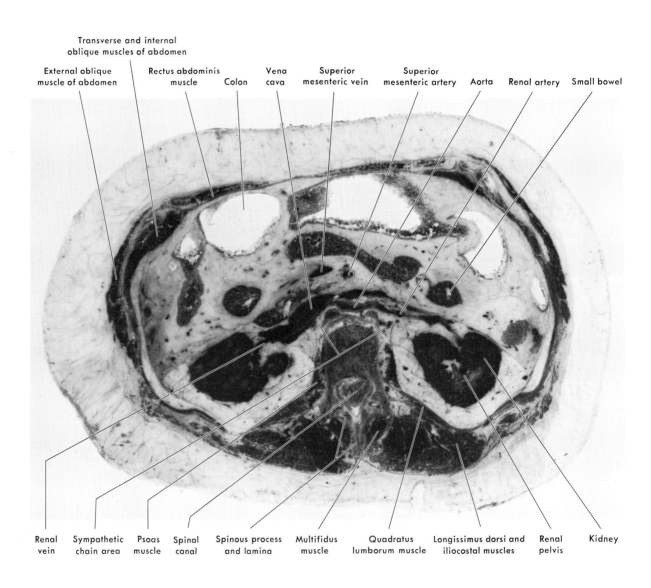

Transverse and internal
oblique muscles of abdomen

External oblique
muscle of abdomen

Rectus abdominis
muscle

Colon

Vena
cava

Superior
mesenteric vein

Superior
mesenteric artery

Aorta

Renal artery

Small bowel

Renal
vein

Sympathetic
chain area

Psoas
muscle

Spinal
canal

Spinous process
and lamina

Multifidus
muscle

Quadratus
lumborum muscle

Longissimus dorsi and
iliocostal muscles

Renal
pelvis

Kidney

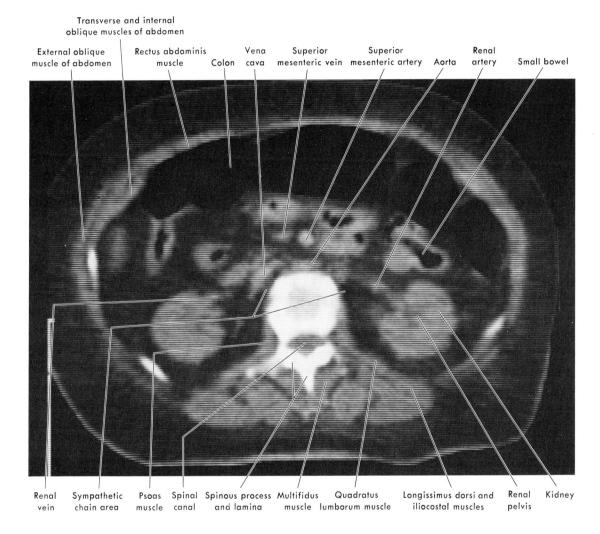

Transverse and internal
oblique muscles of abdomen

External oblique
muscle of abdomen

Rectus abdominis
muscle

Colon

Vena
cava

Superior
mesenteric vein

Superior
mesenteric artery

Aorta

Renal
artery

Small bowel

Renal
vein

Sympathetic
chain area

Psoas
muscle

Spinal
canal

Spinous process
and lamina

Multifidus
muscle

Quadratus
lumborum muscle

Longissimus dorsi and
iliocostal muscles

Renal
pelvis

Kidney

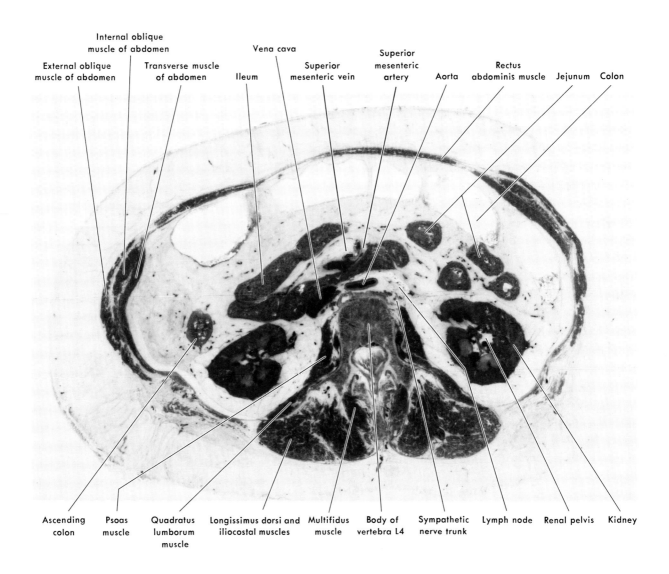

Internal oblique
muscle of abdomen

External oblique
muscle of abdomen

Transverse muscle
of abdomen

Ileum

Vena cava

Superior
mesenteric vein

Superior
mesenteric
artery

Aorta

Rectus
abdominis muscle

Jejunum   Colon

Ascending
colon

Psoas
muscle

Quadratus
lumborum
muscle

Longissimus dorsi and
iliocostal muscles

Multifidus
muscle

Body of
vertebra L4

Sympathetic
nerve trunk

Lymph node   Renal pelvis   Kidney

Internal oblique
muscle of abdomen

External oblique
muscle of abdomen

Transverse muscle
of abdomen

Vena cava

Ileum

Superior
mesenteric vein

Superior
mesenteric
artery

Aorta

Rectus
abdominis muscle

Jejunum

Colon

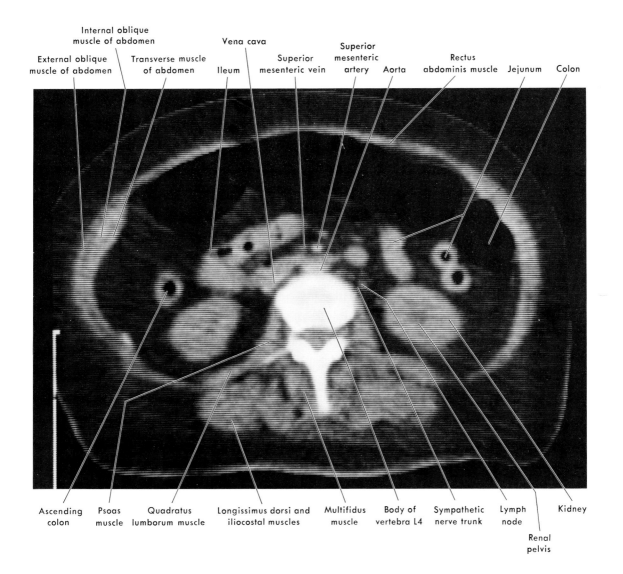

Ascending
colon

Psoas
muscle

Quadratus
lumborum muscle

Longissimus dorsi and
iliocostal muscles

Multifidus
muscle

Body of
vertebra L4

Sympathetic
nerve trunk

Lymph
node

Kidney

Renal
pelvis

Computed tomography of the human body

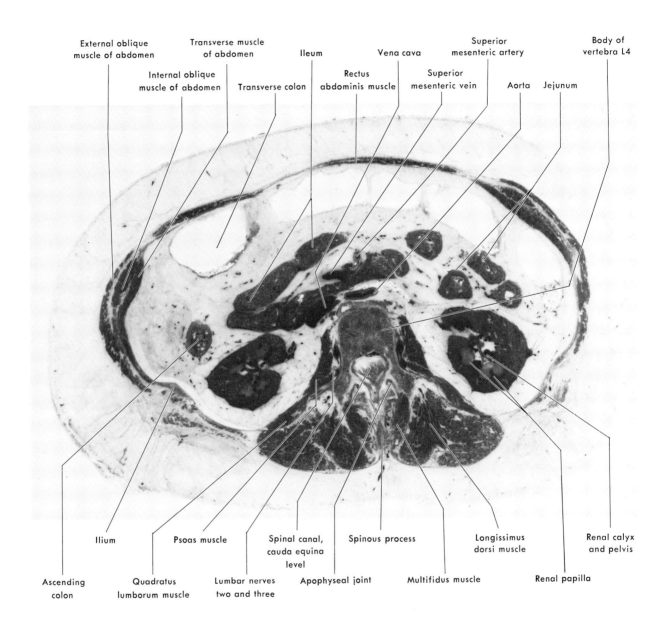

External oblique
muscle of abdomen

Transverse muscle
of abdomen

Ileum

Vena cava

Superior
mesenteric artery

Body of
vertebra L4

Internal oblique
muscle of abdomen

Transverse colon

Rectus
abdominis muscle

Superior
mesenteric vein

Aorta

Jejunum

Ilium

Psoas muscle

Spinal canal,
cauda equina
level

Spinous process

Longissimus
dorsi muscle

Renal calyx
and pelvis

Ascending
colon

Quadratus
lumborum muscle

Lumbar nerves
two and three

Apophyseal joint

Multifidus muscle

Renal papilla

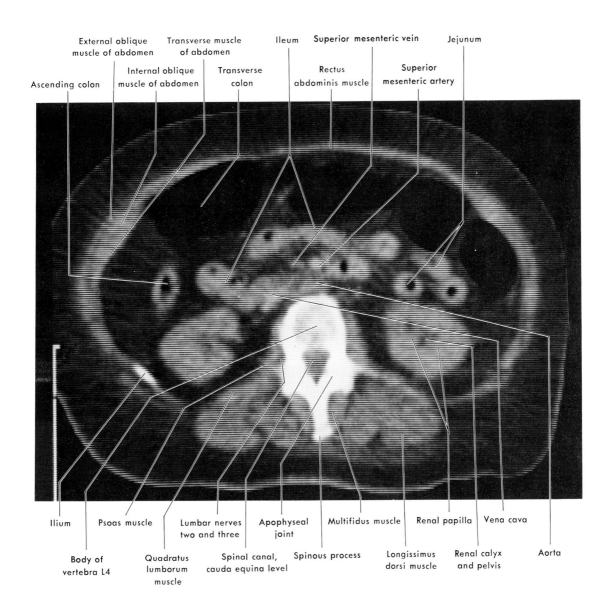

External oblique
muscle of abdomen

Transverse muscle
of abdomen

Ileum   Superior mesenteric vein

Jejunum

Ascending colon

Internal oblique
muscle of abdomen

Transverse
colon

Rectus
abdominis muscle

Superior
mesenteric artery

Ilium   Psoas muscle

Lumbar nerves
two and three

Apophyseal
joint

Multifidus muscle

Renal papilla   Vena cava

Body of
vertebra L4

Quadratus
lumborum
muscle

Spinal canal,
cauda equina level

Spinous process

Longissimus
dorsi muscle

Renal calyx
and pelvis

Aorta

FEMALE

External oblique muscle of abdomen | Internal oblique muscle of abdomen | Transverse muscle of abdomen | Small bowel | Rectus abdominis muscle | Iliac arteries | Iliac veins | Colon | Iliacus muscle | Ilium

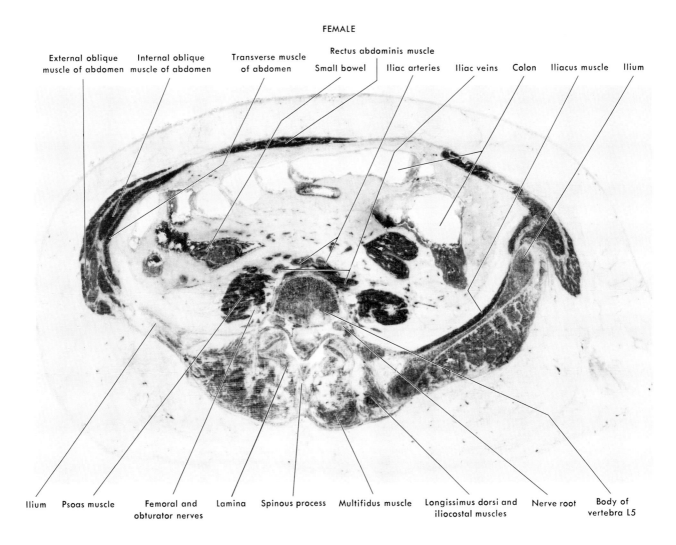

Ilium | Psoas muscle | Femoral and obturator nerves | Lamina | Spinous process | Multifidus muscle | Longissimus dorsi and iliocostal muscles | Nerve root | Body of vertebra L5

FEMALE

External oblique muscle of abdomen   Internal oblique muscle of abdomen   Transverse muscle of abdomen   Rectus abdominis muscle   Iliac arteries   Iliac veins   Colon   Iliacus muscle

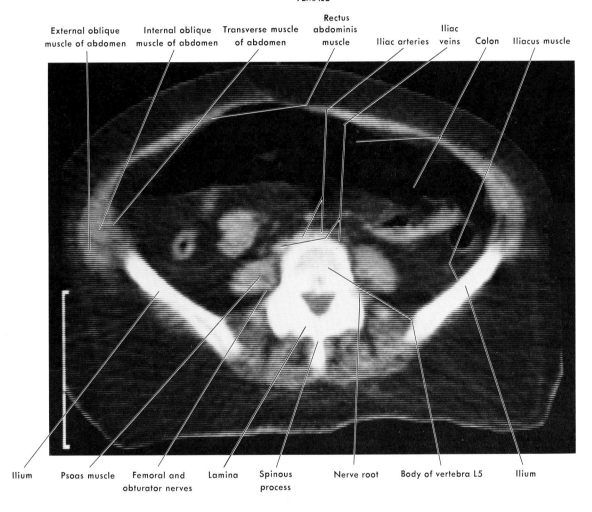

Ilium   Psoas muscle   Femoral and obturator nerves   Lamina   Spinous process   Nerve root   Body of vertebra L5   Ilium

Computed tomography of the human body

FEMALE

Internal and external oblique and transverse muscles of abdomen

Colon

Rectus abdominis muscle

Iliac arteries

Bifurcation of iliac veins

Small bowel

Psoas muscle

Internal and external oblique and transverse muscles of abdomen

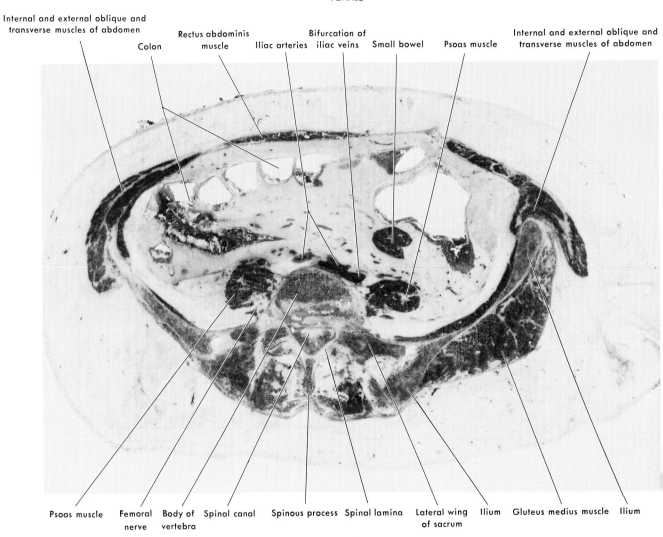

Psoas muscle

Femoral nerve

Body of vertebra

Spinal canal

Spinous process

Spinal lamina

Lateral wing of sacrum

Ilium

Gluteus medius muscle

Ilium

FEMALE

Internal and external oblique and
transverse muscles of abdomen

Iliac arteries

Colon

Bifurcation of
iliac veins

Rectus
abdominis
muscle

Small
bowel

Internal and external oblique and
transverse muscles of abdomen

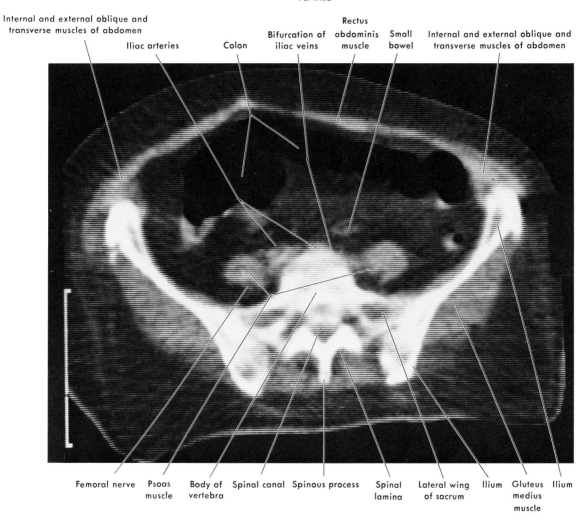

Femoral nerve   Psoas
muscle

Body of
vertebra

Spinal canal   Spinous process

Spinal
lamina

Lateral wing
of sacrum

Ilium

Gluteus
medius
muscle

Ilium

Computed tomography of the human body

FEMALE

Transverse and internal
oblique muscles of abdomen

Gluteus minimus muscle   Colon   Femoral nerve   Rectus abdominis muscle   Iliopsoas muscle   External iliac artery   Gluteus minimus muscle

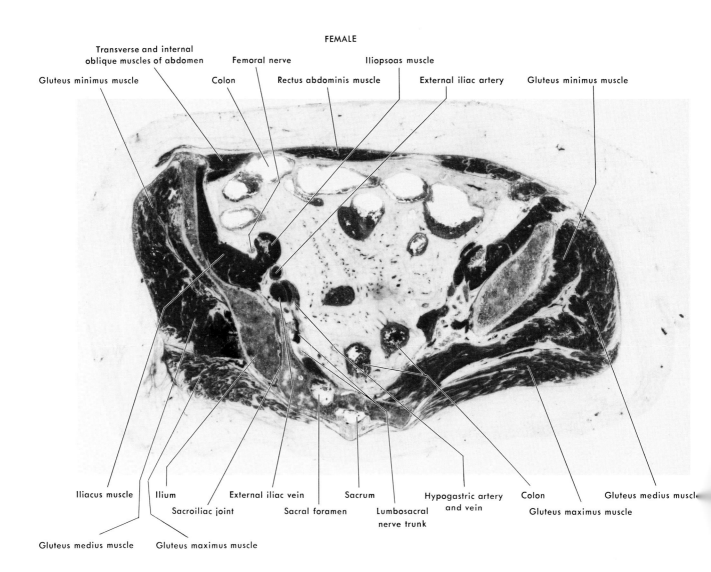

Iliacus muscle   Ilium   External iliac vein   Sacrum   Hypogastric artery   Colon   Gluteus medius muscl

Sacroiliac joint   Sacral foramen   Lumbosacral   and vein   Gluteus maximus muscle

nerve trunk

Gluteus medius muscle   Gluteus maximus muscle

FEMALE

Gluteus minimus muscle

Transverse and internal oblique muscles of abdomen

Iliacus muscle

Femoral nerve

Colon

Rectus abdominis muscle

Iliopsoas muscle

External iliac artery

Hypogastric artery and vein

External iliac vein

Gluteus minimus muscle

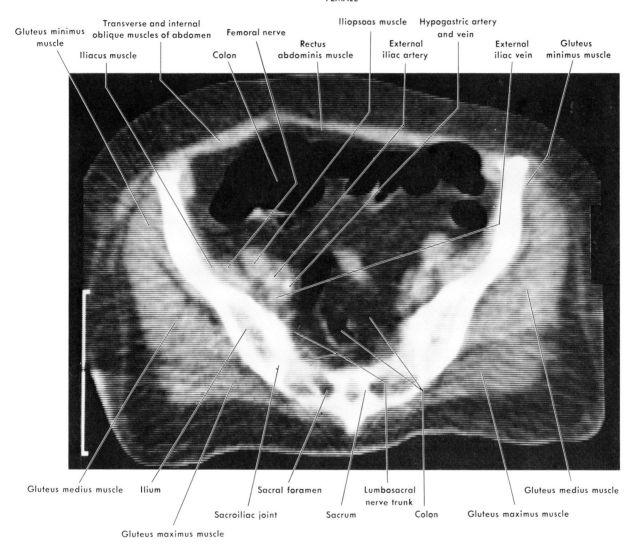

Gluteus medius muscle

Ilium

Gluteus maximus muscle

Sacroiliac joint

Sacral foramen

Sacrum

Lumbosacral nerve trunk

Colon

Gluteus medius muscle

Gluteus maximus muscle

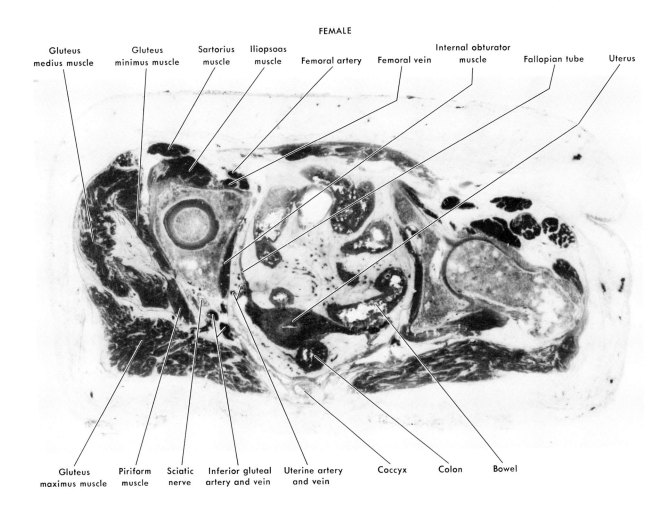

FEMALE

Gluteus medius muscle   Gluteus minimus muscle   Sartorius muscle   Iliopsoas muscle   Femoral artery   Femoral vein   Internal obturator muscle   Fallopian tube   Uterus

Gluteus maximus muscle   Piriform muscle   Sciatic nerve   Inferior gluteal artery and vein   Uterine artery and vein   Coccyx   Colon   Bowel

FEMALE

Gluteus medius muscle

Gluteus minimus muscle

Sartorius muscle

Iliopsoas muscle

Femoral artery

Femoral vein

Internal obturator muscle

Fallopian tube

Uterus

Gluteus maximus muscle

Piriform muscle

Sciatic nerve

Inferior gluteal artery and vein

Uterine artery and vein

Coccyx

Colon

Bowel

Computed tomography of the human body

FEMALE

Tensor fasciae latae muscle
Sartorius muscle
Iliopsoas muscle
Bowel
Superior ramus of pubis
Femoral vein
Femoral artery
Iliopsoas muscle
Sartorius muscle
Rectus femoris muscle
Tensor fasciae latae muscle

Gluteus maximus muscle
Uterus
Coccyx
Fallopian tube
Sciatic nerve
Gluteus minimus muscle
Internal obturator muscle
Gluteus maximus muscle

FEMALE

Tensor fasciae
latae muscle

Sartorius muscle

Iliopsoas muscle

Bowel

Superior ramus
of pubis

Femoral vein

Femoral artery

Iliopsoas muscle

Sartorius muscle

Rectus femoris muscle

Tensor fasciae
latae muscle

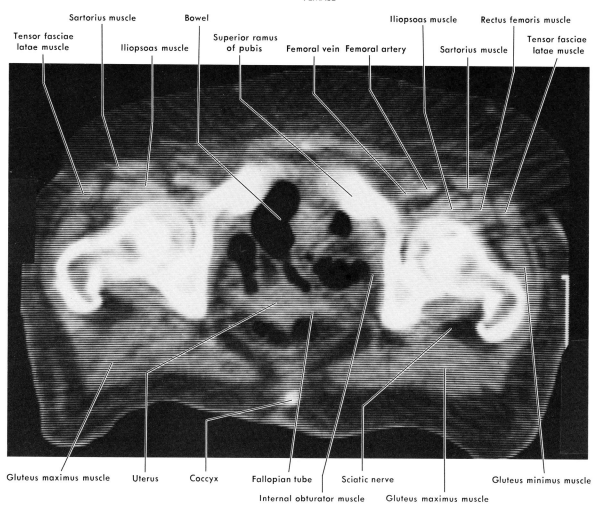

Gluteus maximus muscle

Uterus

Coccyx

Fallopian tube

Internal obturator muscle

Sciatic nerve

Gluteus maximus muscle

Gluteus minimus muscle

FEMALE

Rectus femoris
muscle

Tensor fasciae
latae muscle

Sartorius
muscle

Iliopsoas
muscle

Pubic
bones

Cartilaginous
symphysis

Internal
obturator muscle

External
obturator muscle

Pectineus
muscle

Femoral
vein

Femoral
artery

Femoral
nerve

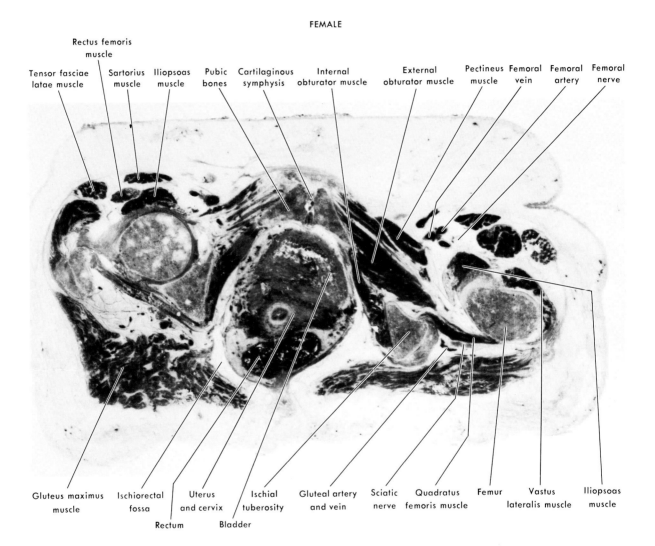

Gluteus maximus
muscle

Ischiorectal
fossa

Uterus
and cervix

Rectum

Ischial
tuberosity

Bladder

Gluteal artery
and vein

Sciatic
nerve

Quadratus
femoris muscle

Femur

Vastus
lateralis muscle

Iliopsoas
muscle

FEMALE

Tensor fasciae
latae muscle

Rectus femoris
muscle

Sartorius
muscle

Iliopsoas
muscle

Pubic
bones

Cartilaginous
symphysis

Internal
obturator muscle

External
obturator muscle

Pectineus
muscle

Femoral
vein

Femoral
artery

Femoral
nerve

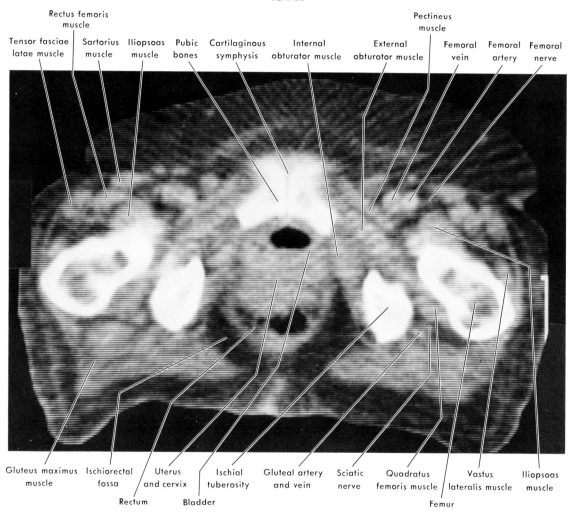

Gluteus maximus
muscle

Ischiorectal
fossa

Uterus
and cervix

Rectum

Ischial
tuberosity

Bladder

Gluteal artery
and vein

Sciatic
nerve

Quadratus
femoris muscle

Femur

Vastus
lateralis muscle

Iliopsoas
muscle

Computed tomography of the human body

FEMALE

Rectus femoris
muscle

Tensor fasciae
latae muscle

Sartorius
muscle

Iliopsoas
muscle

Pubic
bone

Symphysis
pubis

Adductor
longus muscle

External obturator
muscle

Adductor
minimus muscle

Pectineus
muscle

Femoral
vein

Femoral
artery

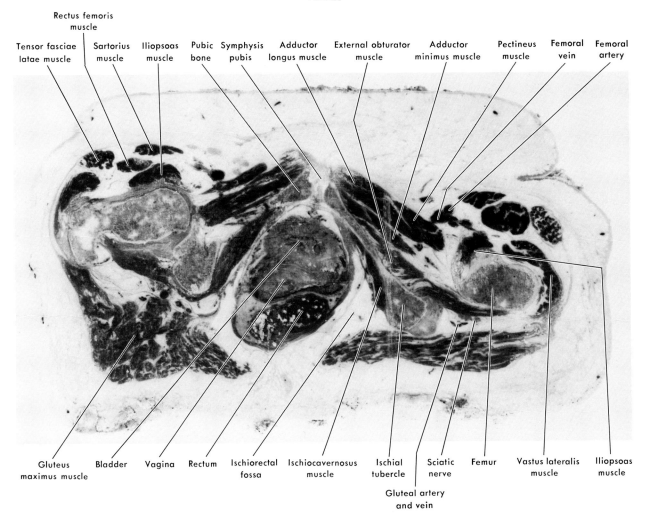

Gluteus
maximus muscle

Bladder

Vagina

Rectum

Ischiorectal
fossa

Ischiocavernosus
muscle

Ischial
tubercle

Sciatic
nerve

Femur

Vastus lateralis
muscle

Iliopsoas
muscle

Gluteal artery
and vein

168

FEMALE

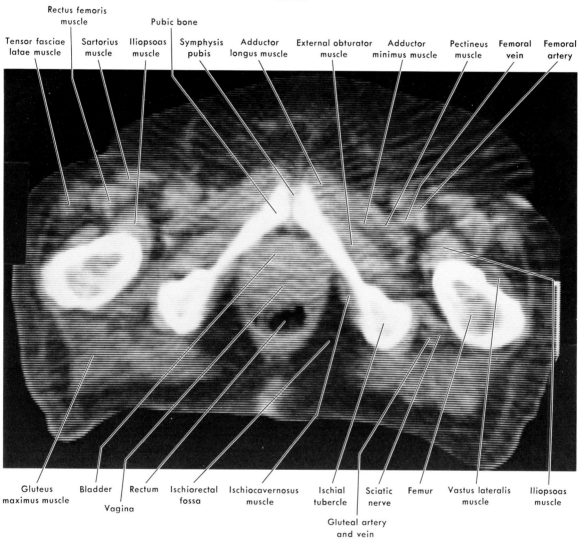

Rectus femoris
muscle

Pubic bone

Tensor fasciae
latae muscle

Sartorius
muscle

Iliopsoas
muscle

Symphysis
pubis

Adductor
longus muscle

External obturator
muscle

Adductor
minimus muscle

Pectineus
muscle

Femoral
vein

Femoral
artery

Gluteus
maximus muscle

Bladder

Vagina

Rectum

Ischiorectal
fossa

Ischiocavernosus
muscle

Ischial
tubercle

Sciatic
nerve

Gluteal artery
and vein

Femur

Vastus lateralis
muscle

Iliopsoas
muscle

Computed tomography of the human body

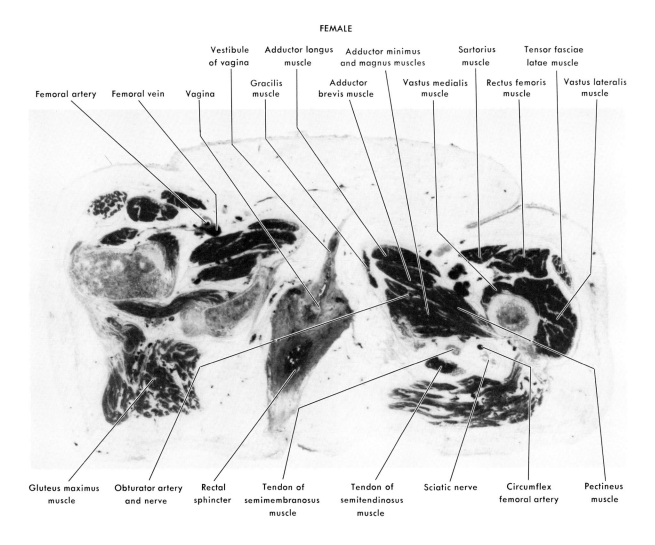

FEMALE

Femoral artery   Femoral vein   Vagina   Vestibule of vagina   Gracilis muscle   Adductor longus muscle   Adductor brevis muscle   Adductor minimus and magnus muscles   Vastus medialis muscle   Sartorius muscle   Rectus femoris muscle   Tensor fasciae latae muscle   Vastus lateralis muscle

Gluteus maximus muscle   Obturator artery and nerve   Rectal sphincter   Tendon of semimembranosus muscle   Tendon of semitendinosus muscle   Sciatic nerve   Circumflex femoral artery   Pectineus muscle

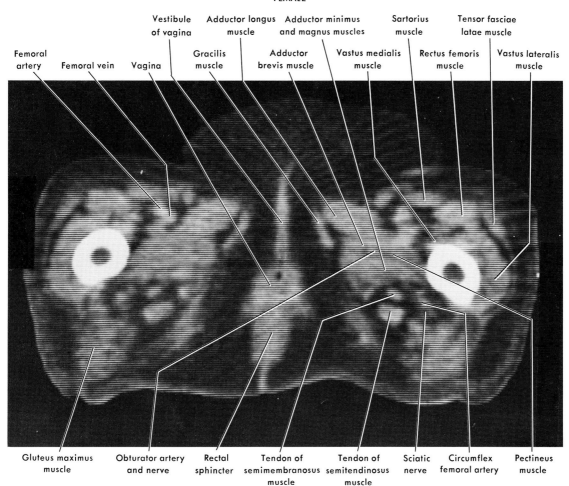

FEMALE

Vestibule of vagina • Adductor longus muscle • Adductor minimus and magnus muscles • Sartorius muscle • Tensor fasciae latae muscle

Femoral artery • Femoral vein • Vagina • Gracilis muscle • Adductor brevis muscle • Vastus medialis muscle • Rectus femoris muscle • Vastus lateralis muscle

Gluteus maximus muscle • Obturator artery and nerve • Rectal sphincter • Tendon of semimembranosus muscle • Tendon of semitendinosus muscle • Sciatic nerve • Circumflex femoral artery • Pectineus muscle

Computed tomography of the human body

MALE

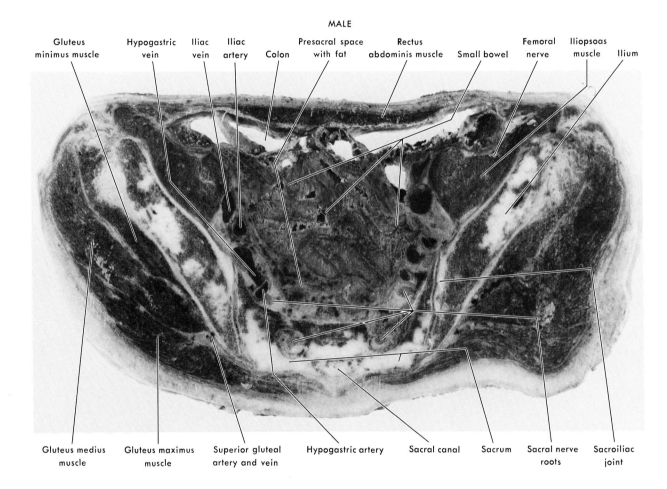

Gluteus minimus muscle | Hypogastric vein | Iliac vein | Iliac artery | Colon | Presacral space with fat | Rectus abdominis muscle | Small bowel | Femoral nerve | Iliopsoas muscle | Ilium

Gluteus medius muscle | Gluteus maximus muscle | Superior gluteal artery and vein | Hypogastric artery | Sacral canal | Sacrum | Sacral nerve roots | Sacroiliac joint

MALE

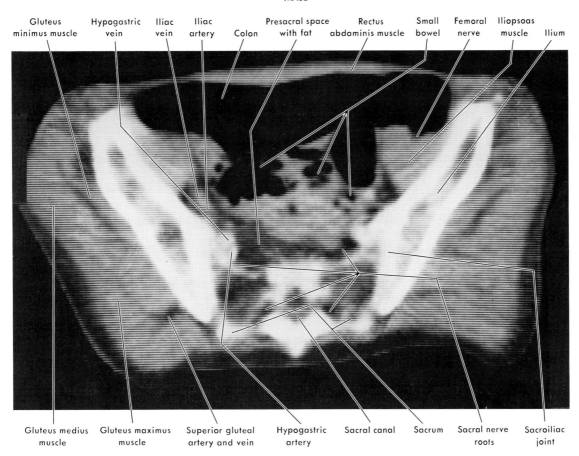

Gluteus minimus muscle · Hypogastric vein · Iliac vein · Iliac artery · Colon · Presacral space with fat · Rectus abdominis muscle · Small bowel · Femoral nerve · Iliopsoas muscle · Ilium

Gluteus medius muscle · Gluteus maximus muscle · Superior gluteal artery and vein · Hypogastric artery · Sacral canal · Sacrum · Sacral nerve roots · Sacroiliac joint

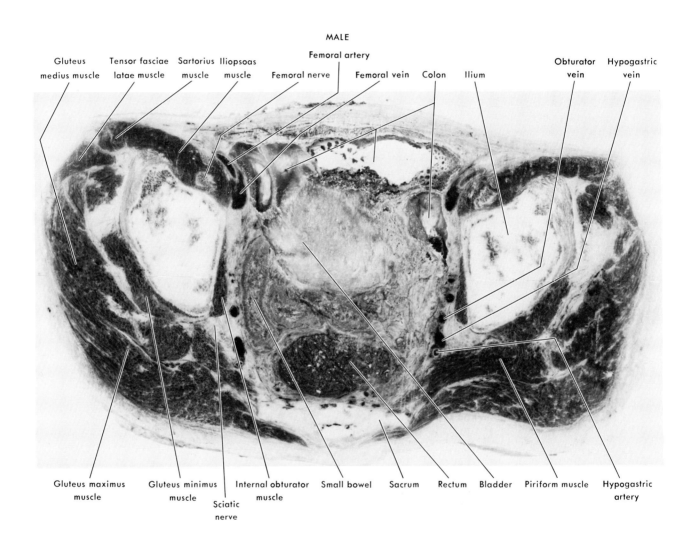

MALE

Gluteus medius muscle · Tensor fasciae latae muscle · Sartorius muscle · Iliopsoas muscle · Femoral nerve · Femoral artery · Femoral vein · Colon · Ilium · Obturator vein · Hypogastric vein

Gluteus maximus muscle · Gluteus minimus muscle · Sciatic nerve · Internal obturator muscle · Small bowel · Sacrum · Rectum · Bladder · Piriform muscle · Hypogastric artery

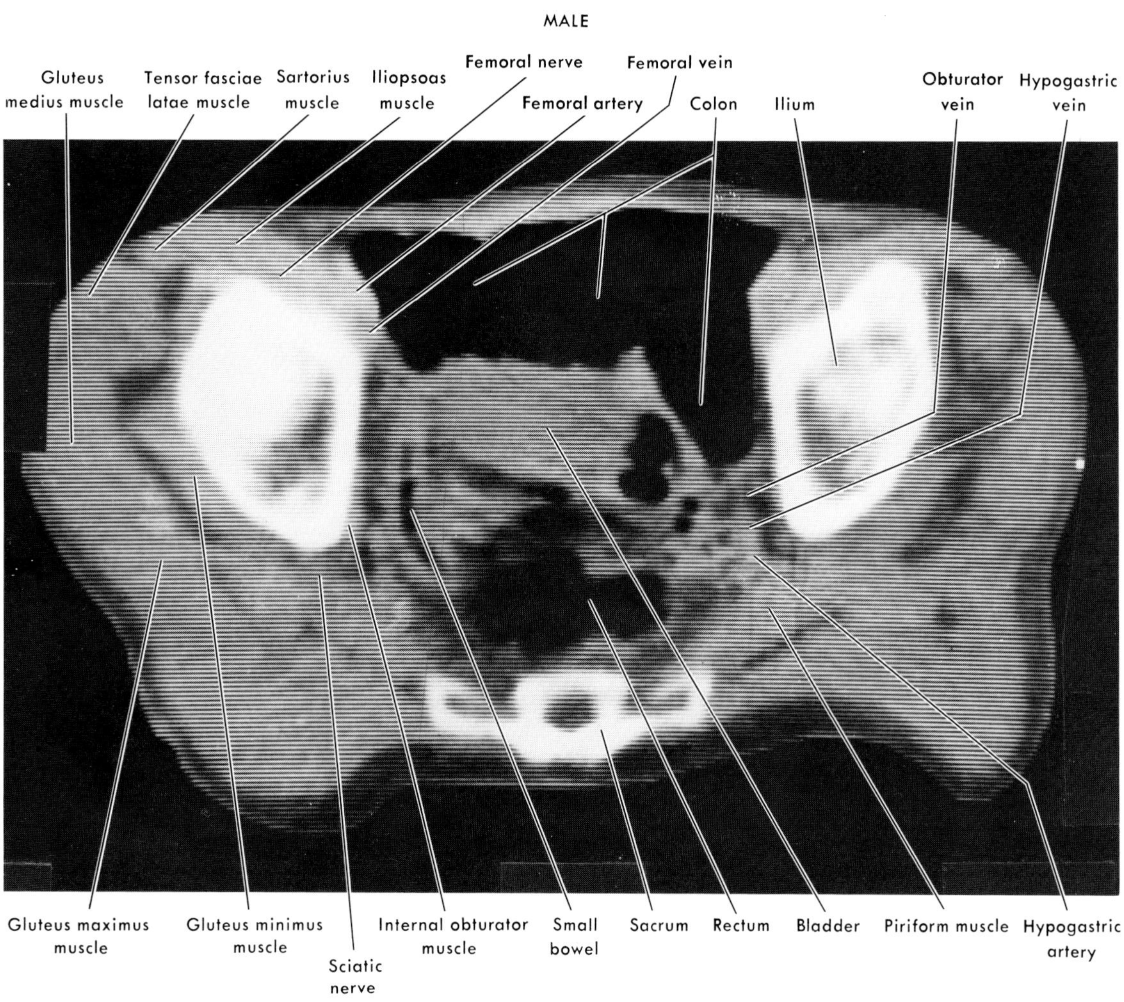

MALE

Gluteus
medius muscle

Tensor fasciae
latae muscle

Sartorius
muscle

Iliopsoas
muscle

Femoral nerve

Femoral artery

Femoral vein

Colon

Ilium

Obturator
vein

Hypogastric
vein

Gluteus maximus
muscle

Gluteus minimus
muscle

Sciatic
nerve

Internal obturator
muscle

Small
bowel

Sacrum

Rectum

Bladder

Piriform muscle

Hypogastric
artery

Computed tomography of the human body

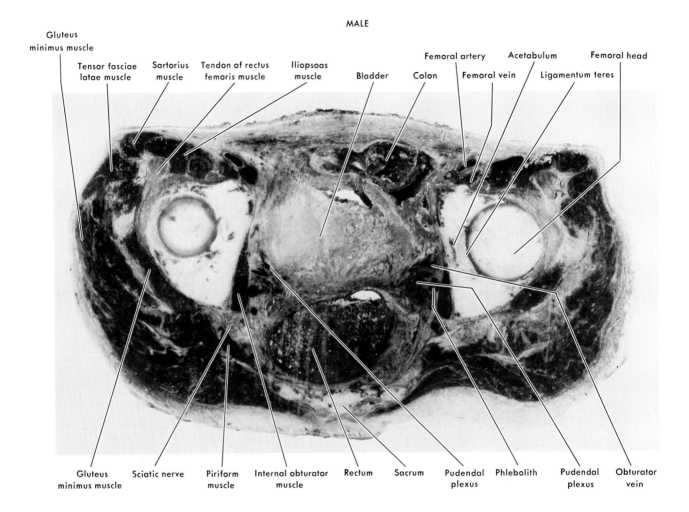

Gluteus
minimus muscle

Tensor fasciae
latae muscle

Sartorius
muscle

Tendon of rectus
femoris muscle

Iliopsoas
muscle

Bladder

Colon

Femoral artery

Femoral vein

Acetabulum

Ligamentum teres

Femoral head

Gluteus
minimus muscle

Sciatic nerve

Piriform
muscle

Internal obturator
muscle

Rectum

Sacrum

Pudendal
plexus

Phlebolith

Pudendal
plexus

Obturator
vein

176

MALE

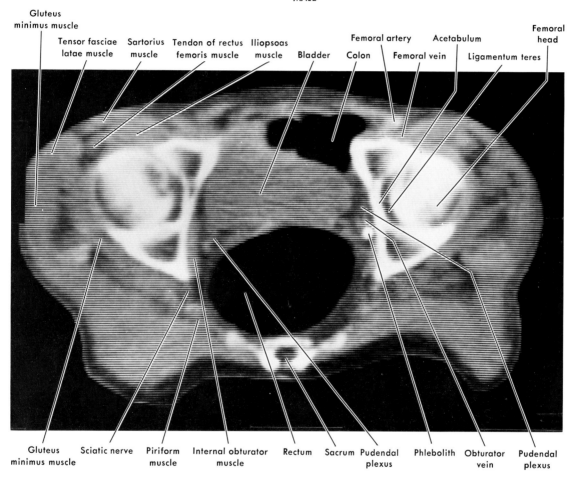

Gluteus
minimus muscle

Tensor fasciae   Sartorius   Tendon of rectus   Iliopsoas   Femoral artery   Acetabulum   Femoral
latae muscle   muscle   femoris muscle   muscle   Bladder   Colon   Femoral vein   Ligamentum teres   head

Gluteus   Sciatic nerve   Piriform   Internal obturator   Rectum   Sacrum   Pudendal   Phlebolith   Obturator   Pudendal
minimus muscle   muscle   muscle   plexus   vein   plexus

Computed tomography of the human body

MALE

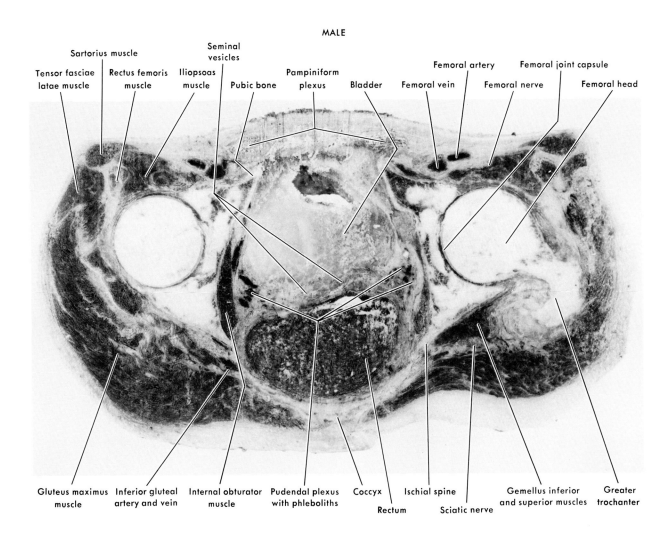

MALE

Tensor fasciae latae muscle · Sartorius muscle · Rectus femoris muscle · Iliopsoas muscle · Pubic bone · Seminal vesicles · Pampiniform plexus · Bladder · Femoral vein · Femoral artery · Femoral nerve · Femoral joint capsule · Femoral head

Gluteus maximus muscle · Inferior gluteal artery and vein · Internal obturator muscle · Pudendal plexus with phleboliths · Coccyx · Rectum · Ischial spine · Sciatic nerve · Gemellus inferior and superior muscles · Greater trochanter

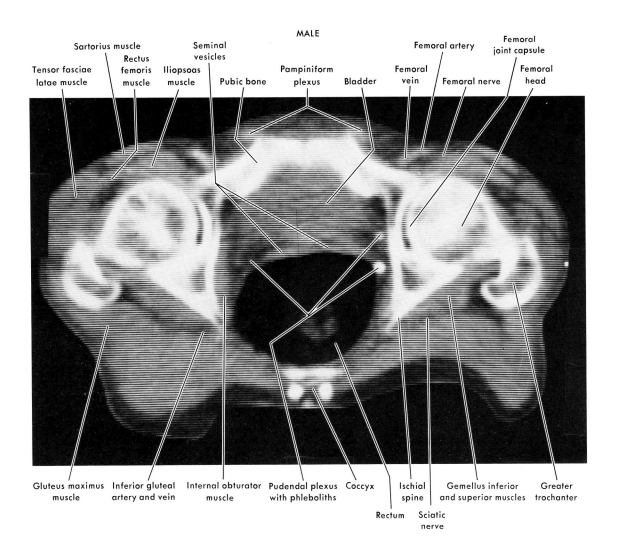

MALE

Tensor fasciae latae muscle

Sartorius muscle

Rectus femoris muscle

Iliopsoas muscle

Seminal vesicles

Pubic bone

Pampiniform plexus

Bladder

Femoral vein

Femoral artery

Femoral nerve

Femoral joint capsule

Femoral head

Gluteus maximus muscle

Inferior gluteal artery and vein

Internal obturator muscle

Pudendal plexus with phleboliths

Coccyx

Rectum

Ischial spine

Sciatic nerve

Gemellus inferior and superior muscles

Greater trochanter

Computed tomography of the human body

MALE

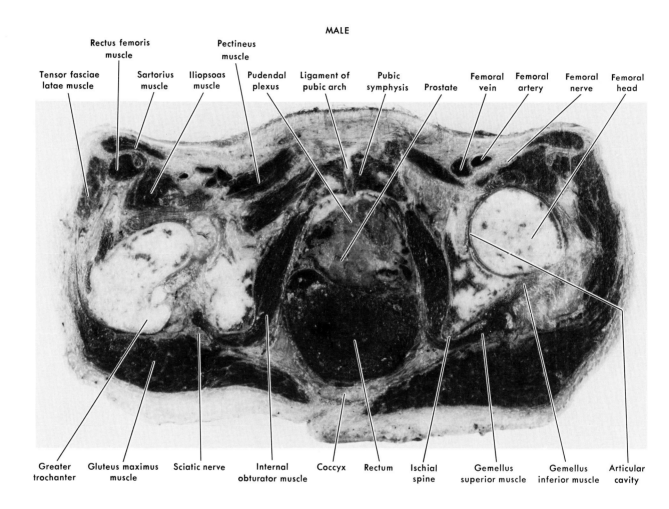

Tensor fasciae latae muscle · Rectus femoris muscle · Sartorius muscle · Iliopsoas muscle · Pectineus muscle · Pudendal plexus · Ligament of pubic arch · Pubic symphysis · Prostate · Femoral vein · Femoral artery · Femoral nerve · Femoral head

Greater trochanter · Gluteus maximus muscle · Sciatic nerve · Internal obturator muscle · Coccyx · Rectum · Ischial spine · Gemellus superior muscle · Gemellus inferior muscle · Articular cavity

MALE

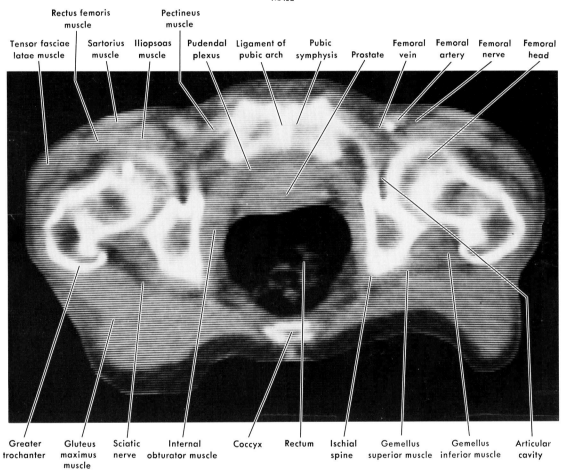

Rectus femoris muscle

Pectineus muscle

Tensor fasciae latae muscle

Sartorius muscle

Iliopsoas muscle

Pudendal plexus

Ligament of pubic arch

Pubic symphysis

Prostate

Femoral vein

Femoral artery

Femoral nerve

Femoral head

Greater trochanter

Gluteus maximus muscle

Sciatic nerve

Internal obturator muscle

Coccyx

Rectum

Ischial spine

Gemellus superior muscle

Gemellus inferior muscle

Articular cavity

MALE

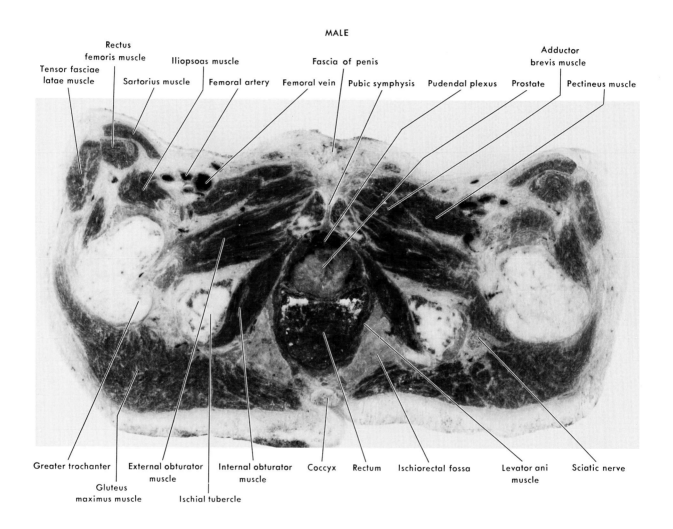

Tensor fasciae latae muscle — Rectus femoris muscle — Sartorius muscle — Iliopsoas muscle — Femoral artery — Femoral vein — Fascia of penis — Pubic symphysis — Pudendal plexus — Prostate — Adductor brevis muscle — Pectineus muscle

Greater trochanter — Gluteus maximus muscle — External obturator muscle — Ischial tubercle — Internal obturator muscle — Coccyx — Rectum — Ischiorectal fossa — Levator ani muscle — Sciatic nerve

MALE

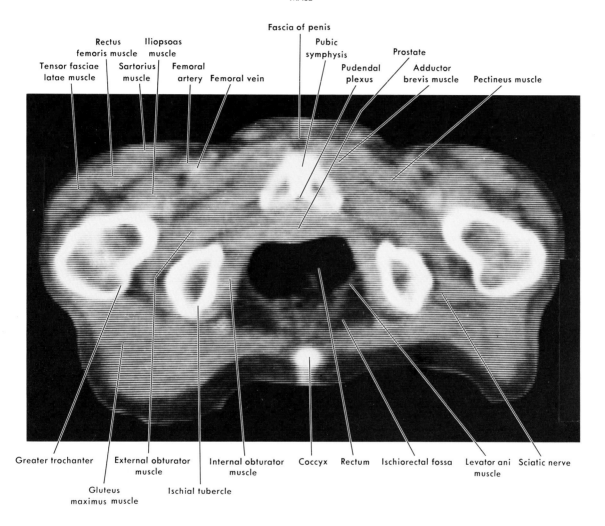

Tensor fasciae latae muscle · Rectus femoris muscle · Sartorius muscle · Iliopsoas muscle · Femoral artery · Femoral vein · Fascia of penis · Pubic symphysis · Pudendal plexus · Prostate · Adductor brevis muscle · Pectineus muscle

Greater trochanter · Gluteus maximus muscle · External obturator muscle · Ischial tubercle · Internal obturator muscle · Coccyx · Rectum · Ischiorectal fossa · Levator ani muscle · Sciatic nerve

Computed tomography of the human body

MALE

Tensor fasciae latae muscle

Vastus lateralis muscle

Rectus femoris muscle

Sartorius muscle

Pectineus muscle

Adductor brevis muscle

Adductor minimus muscle

External obturator muscle

Adductor longus muscle

Pampiniform plexus

Penis

Prostate

Ischiocavernosus muscle

Femoral vein

Femoral artery

Femoral nerve

Deep femoral artery

Iliopsoas muscle

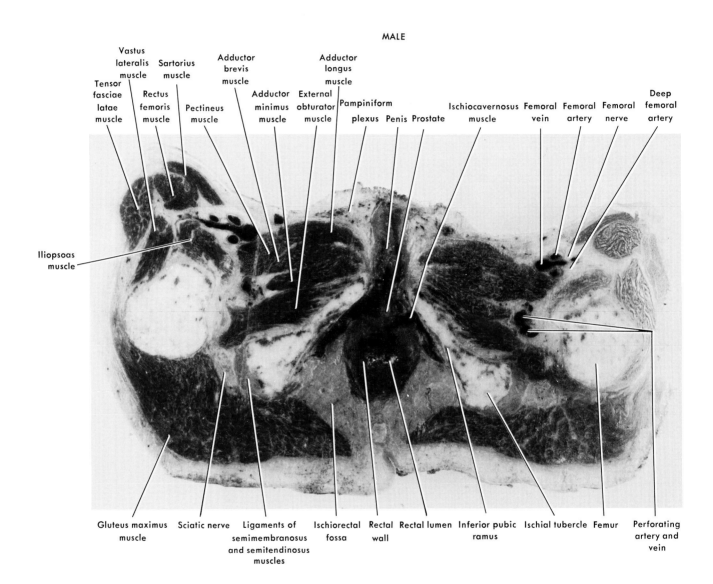

Gluteus maximus muscle

Sciatic nerve

Ligaments of semimembranosus and semitendinosus muscles

Ischiorectal fossa

Rectal wall

Rectal lumen

Inferior pubic ramus

Ischial tubercle

Femur

Perforating artery and vein

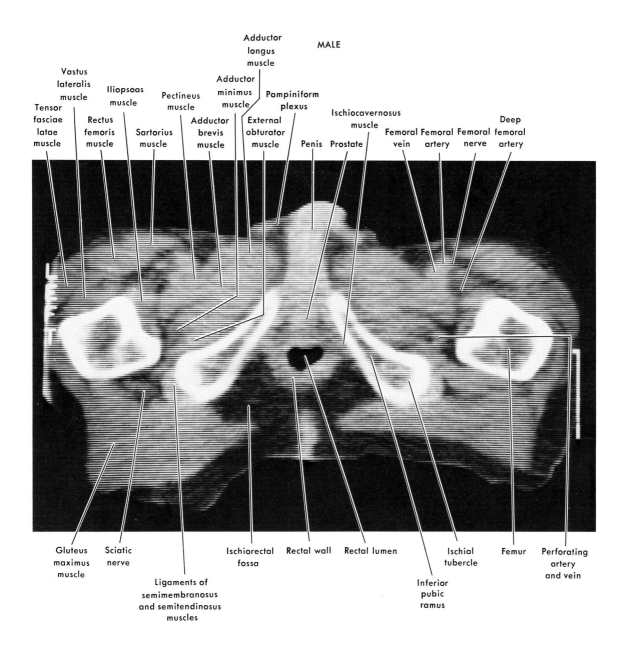

MALE

Adductor longus muscle

Vastus lateralis muscle

Adductor minimus muscle

Iliopsoas muscle

Pampiniform plexus

Pectineus muscle

Tensor fasciae latae muscle

Rectus femoris muscle

Adductor brevis muscle

External obturator muscle

Ischiocavernosus muscle

Deep femoral artery

Sartorius muscle

Penis

Prostate

Femoral vein

Femoral artery

Femoral nerve

Gluteus maximus muscle

Sciatic nerve

Ischiorectal fossa

Rectal wall

Rectal lumen

Ischial tubercle

Femur

Perforating artery and vein

Ligaments of semimembranosus and semitendinosus muscles

Inferior pubic ramus

Computed tomography of the human body

MALE

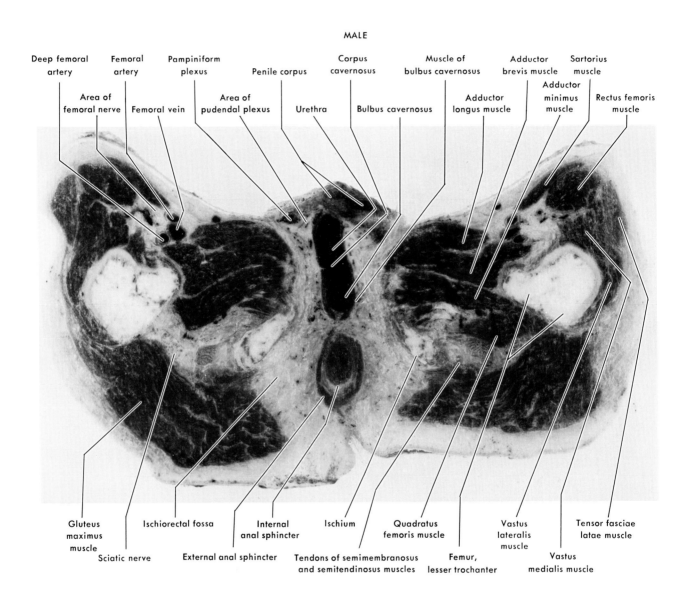

Deep femoral artery · Femoral artery · Pampiniform plexus · Penile corpus · Corpus cavernosus · Muscle of bulbus cavernosus · Adductor brevis muscle · Sartorius muscle

Area of femoral nerve · Femoral vein · Area of pudendal plexus · Urethra · Bulbus cavernosus · Adductor longus muscle · Adductor minimus muscle · Rectus femoris muscle

Gluteus maximus muscle · Ischiorectal fossa · Internal anal sphincter · Ischium · Quadratus femoris muscle · Vastus lateralis muscle · Tensor fasciae latae muscle

Sciatic nerve · External anal sphincter · Tendons of semimembranosus and semitendinosus muscles · Femur, lesser trochanter · Vastus medialis muscle

MALE

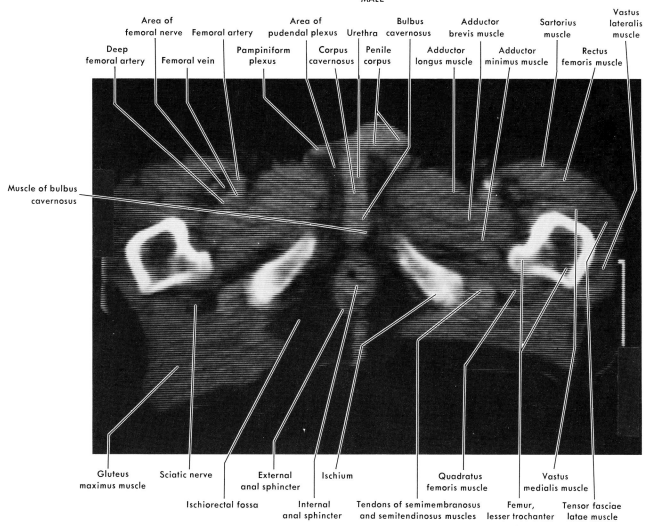

Deep femoral artery · Area of femoral nerve · Femoral artery · Femoral vein · Pampiniform plexus · Area of pudendal plexus · Corpus cavernosus · Urethra · Penile corpus · Bulbus cavernosus · Adductor longus muscle · Adductor brevis muscle · Adductor minimus muscle · Sartorius muscle · Rectus femoris muscle · Vastus lateralis muscle

Muscle of bulbus cavernosus

Gluteus maximus muscle · Sciatic nerve · Ischiorectal fossa · External anal sphincter · Internal anal sphincter · Ischium · Tendons of semimembranosus and semitendinosus muscles · Quadratus femoris muscle · Femur, lesser trochanter · Vastus medialis muscle · Tensor fasciae latae muscle

Computed tomography of the human body

MALE

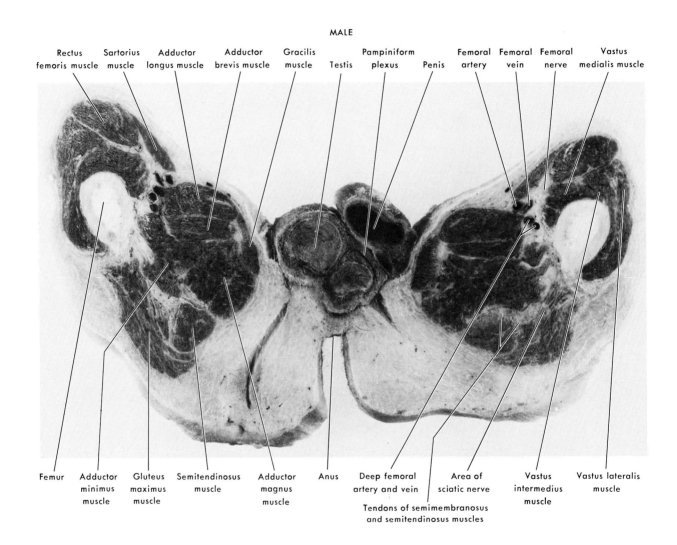

Rectus femoris muscle · Sartorius muscle · Adductor longus muscle · Adductor brevis muscle · Gracilis muscle · Testis · Pampiniform plexus · Penis · Femoral artery · Femoral vein · Femoral nerve · Vastus medialis muscle

Femur · Adductor minimus muscle · Gluteus maximus muscle · Semitendinosus muscle · Adductor magnus muscle · Anus · Deep femoral artery and vein · Area of sciatic nerve · Vastus intermedius muscle · Vastus lateralis muscle

Tendons of semimembranosus and semitendinosus muscles

MALE

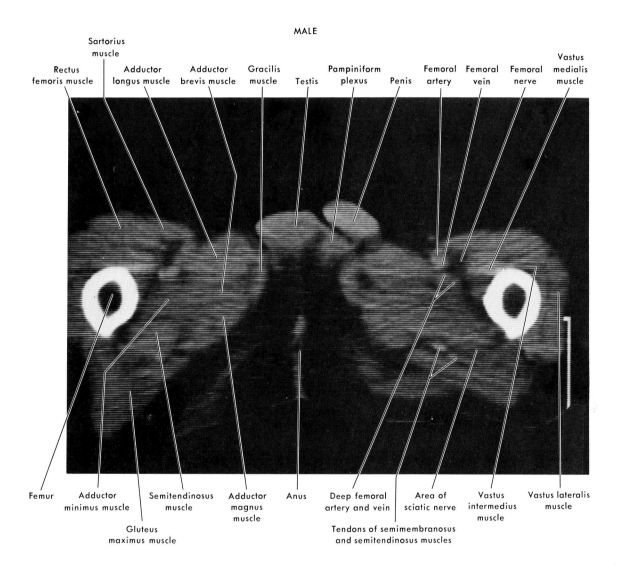

Sartorius
muscle

Rectus
femoris muscle

Adductor
longus muscle

Adductor
brevis muscle

Gracilis
muscle

Testis

Pampiniform
plexus

Penis

Femoral
artery

Femoral
vein

Femoral
nerve

Vastus
medialis
muscle

Femur

Adductor
minimus muscle

Semitendinosus
muscle

Gluteus
maximus muscle

Adductor
magnus
muscle

Anus

Deep femoral
artery and vein

Tendons of semimembranosus
and semitendinosus muscles

Area of
sciatic nerve

Vastus
intermedius
muscle

Vastus lateralis
muscle

INDEX

Index

Index

Index